Lodewijk Brunt / Brigit

Worlds of Sl

Lodewijk Brunt / Brigitte Steger (eds)

Worlds of Sleep

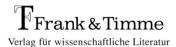

Frank & Timme

Verlag für wissenschaftliche Literatur

Book cover: Co-sleeping during a week-long festival.
Bayan, Lombok Island, Indonesia.
Photo by Brigitte Steger.

Financial support received from Japanese Studies funds
in the Department of East Asian Studies,
University of Cambridge, gratefully acknowledged.

ISBN 978-3-86596-173-0

Herstellung durch das atelier eilenberger, Leipzig.
Printed in Germany.
Gedruckt auf säurefreiem, alterungsbeständigem Papier.

www.frank-timme.de

Acknowledgements

Earlier versions of the contributions in this book have been presented during the workshop 'New Directions in the Social and Cultural Study of Sleep', organised at the University of Vienna from 7 to 9 June 2007.

For financial support we thank the Dean of the Faculty of Philological and Cultural Studies and the Rector of the University of Vienna, the Austrian Ministry of Science and Research, and the Austrian Research Association (ÖFG).

The Department of East Asian Studies, University of Vienna provided us with their fantastic infrastructure, and we thank esp. Anita Szemethy for her support, Bernhard Seidl for lending us his time and skills in designing invitations, and all the colleagues who were willing to relocate their classes. Katja Gutenberger helped us to organise the workshop and made sure that all our participants were kept properly awake with coffee and vitamins.

We are also indebted to the wine maker Weingut Mathias und Regina Schüller in the village of Rauchenwarth, east of Vienna, who generously sponsored a wine tasting at our opening reception.

We are grateful for the printing support for this book which was generously provided by Japanese Studies funds in the Department of East Asian Studies at the University of Cambridge, UK.

Brigitte Steger and Lodewijk Brunt

Nota bene:
All names appear in natural order; that is to say that Chinese and Japanese surnames are followed by given names.

Table of Contents

Introduction 9
LODEWIJK BRUNT AND BRIGITTE STEGER

Dangerous Doze: Sleep and Vulnerability in
Medieval German Literature 31
GABRIELE KLUG

The Suburbs of Eternity: On Visionaries and Miraculous Sleepers 53
ROBERT S. COX

Beds Visible and Invisible:
Hygiene, Morals and Status in Dutch Bedrooms............................. 75
ILEEN MONTIJN

A Bed for Two? Gender Differences in the Reactions to Pair-sleep 93
GERHARD KLOESCH AND JOHN P. DITTAMI

Conflicting Sleep Demands:
Parents and Young People in UK Households................................. 105
SUSAN VENN AND SARA ARBER

Women's Sleep in Italy: The Influence of Caregiving Roles........................ 131
EMANUELA BIANCHERA AND SARA ARBER

Sote hue log: In and Out of Sleep in India 153
LODEWIJK BRUNT

'It's Bedtime' in the World's Urban Middle Classes:
Children, Families and Sleep 175
EYAL BEN-ARI

Sleeping as a Refuge? Embodied Vulnerability and Corporeal
Security during Refugees' Sleep at the Thai-Burma Border 193
PIA VOGLER

'Early to Rise': Making the Japanese Healthy, Wealthy,
Wise, Virtuous, and Beautiful 211
BRIGITTE STEGER

Authors.. 237

Index 241

© Frank & Timme   Verlag für wissenschaftliche Literatur

Introduction

LODEWIJK BRUNT AND BRIGITTE STEGER

Sleep has moved centre stage. Hardly a day goes by that sleep does not figure prominently in newspaper and magazine articles, radio and TV programmes, and internet news. It is acceptable to talk of sleep deprivation, co-sleeping, and daytime fatigue; 'power napping' has become a strategic management method for improving people's performance and commitment at work.

In January 2001 we organised a workshop on 'Sleep and the Night in Asia and the West' (Steger and Brunt 2003). At the time we were hard pressed to find any publications on the social and cultural aspects of 'the dark side of life'. In 2007, we organised a follow-up workshop, 'New Directions in the Social and Cultural Study of Sleep' (Vienna, 6 to 9 June 2007), and the picture had changed completely. This sudden attention towards sleep in the humanities and social sciences was triggered by a growing public interest in sleep, which in turn is fed by an extensive academic engagement; scientific sleep research is booming. Sleep labs are being established everywhere and sleep consultants advise not only individuals but also companies. Sleep has become big business.

In an article in a *New York Times* series on sleep (18 November 2007), journalist Jon Moallem remarks that the hallmark of the '1980s power broker' was someone boosting his or her strength and success with a mere few hours of sleep at night. In this day and age, sleep is taken much more seriously. 'Sleep may finally be claiming its place beside diet and exercise as both a critical health issue and a niche for profitable consumer products'. Moallem also estimates that the new American '*sleeponomics*' amounts to a business of over 20 billion US dollars annually. This includes everything from the more than one thousand accredited sleep clinics to innumerable over-the-counter and herbal sleep aides, how-to books and sleep-inducing gadgets and talismans. Moallem went to visit the ZEA sleep sanctuary – a luxury sleep store in Minnesota. He found light-therapy visors, a Zen alarm clock, and a Mumbasa majesty mosquito net in addition to a pair of noise-blocking earplugs going for six hundred dollars a set. Moreover, the store had sixteen varieties of mattresses and thirty different kinds of pillows.

But this is small change compared to the sleeping-pill business. In 2006 nearly fifty million prescriptions were made out – over a fifty percent increase compared to 2001. We are speaking about a four-billion-dollar enterprise that has practically doubled in less than five years. Moallem concludes that the success not only indicates that 'we have an increasingly urgent craving for sleep, but also that many of us have apparently forgotten how to do it altogether' (Moallem 2007).

Pharmacology offers drugs that reputedly enhance performance by keeping people alert and organising their sleep more efficiently. The company Cephalon has a reputation for its Modafinil drug, originally prescribed for the treatment of narcolepsy. The drug is known as a 'wakefulness-promoting agent' and, consequently, is promoted as a stimulant for 'alertness', but also for ADHD. An alarming number of students and truck drivers are taking such drugs (often bought through websites) to enhance their cognitive performance and alertness (Hibbert 2007).

With the explosion in knowledge about the mechanisms and functions of sleep, people – especially in the US, but also elsewhere in the world – are increasingly held responsible for ensuring a good night's sleep and daytime alertness. The American National Sleep Foundation urges us to improve our knowledge and be watchful. On their website they ask questions such as: 'Is insomnia keeping you awake?', 'What do you know about sleep apnea?', 'What do you know about the restless-leg syndrome?', 'Am I getting good sleep?', 'Do I have a sleep disorder?', 'Why is sleep important?', and 'What is the connection between sleep and age?'

In the past, it was common for people to mention discomfort related to sleep or daytime fatigue when consulting their doctor for pain, high blood pressure or depression. However, sleep problems were almost never thought of as an illness, per se. This has changed. The phenomenon of sleep and the environment for sleep has become medicalised. Physicians have strong opinions about 'normal' and/or 'healthy' sleep and they have abundant advice on how to obtain it: at what time people should go to bed, at what time they have to get up, and how long they are supposed to sleep. What kind of beds guarantee people a good and wholesome sleep, what kinds of mattresses, what sorts of pillows (if at all), and what kind of bed clothing? Prescribed are: more jogging, less drinking, going to bed earlier, and avoiding stressful encounters. 'Power napping' and *inemuri* (a Japanese term for napping in trains, during meetings, concerts and lectures; cf. Steger 2006; 2007) are now being taught in seminars on relaxation, performance enhancement and slow living.

The discovery of REM sleep in 1953 is generally regarded as the beginning of modern sleep research, but prior to the 1990s only a few people and institutions thought it worthwhile to spend time and money on sleep. The situation has changed entirely. Most sleep research is conducted in the US. New findings are most willingly embraced there and the National Science Foundation and many ministries and private companies are involved in sleep research. Europe and Japan follow in their research efforts in the field. The Japanese government has financed six years (1996–2002) of intensive sleep research involving almost one hundred researchers, and more publications – including new academic journals devoted entirely to the issue – have become available (Hayaishi 2004). The vanguard of medical and biological sleep research, however, has always been the military (Takada 1993: 66). With improved night-vision and other technology as well as the possibility to relocate large numbers of troops within a short time, the need for the enhancement of soldiers' and commanders' bodies and minds has made sleep research an imperative for modern militaries (Ben-Ari 2003). Indeed, as Gerhard Kloesch asserted during the Vienna workshop on New Directions in the Social and Cultural Study of Sleep, rather than being motivated by the investigators' interest or by social needs, research on the effects of certain pills and substances is often initiated (and financed) by the pharmaceutical industry. They want to find civil applications for their products in order to increase their profits for their sometimes high investments in military sleep research.

Sleep has also become a subject of direct government control. In January 2006, the Spanish government – similar to the Chinese some twenty years earlier (cf. Li 2003) – reduced the lunch break for government officials. This regulation prohibits officials from taking a siesta, but instead, it is argued, they have more quality time for their children in the evening. Spanish time schedules, of course, have now been synchronised with the rest of Europe. The new South Korean prime minister, Lee Myung-bak, has been known to rise at 4.30 a.m. every morning for many years (Wu and Chang 2008). He was quick to re-schedule cabinet meetings at 8 a.m. (instead of 9) and the ministerial reports to the president at 7.30 a.m., which for many of the lower-ranking officials means that they have to start their day in the office at 5 a.m.; without compensation, of course (Shin 2008). This echoes Mao Zedong's scheduling of meetings; but since he had a 28-hour circadian rhythm rather than a 24-hour one, his officials had to show up at any time, day or night, whenever Mao felt like getting some work done (Li 2003: 48). Governments do not always reduce the sleep of their workers. The constitution of Mao's China guaranteed 'working people the right to rest' (Li 2003: 48), which translated into a three-hour lunch break including a widespread habit of midday napping. And the state of Minnesota has postponed the start of the school day by one hour, based on research results indicating that school children do not learn efficiently before 9 a.m. (Wolf-Meyer 2007).

Along with the pharmaceutical industry, other branches of the sleep industry are also developing rapidly. Montijn (in this volume) refers to the successful Dutch firm Auping, which not only produces beds, but also mattresses, cupboards, pillows and all kinds of sheets and accessories including bedside lights, night drawers, dress boys, footstools and backdrops. Their beds cost thousands of euros – some models over ten thousand. Some bedding elements are produced by separate industries, such as pillows, bed linens and mattresses. Moreover, just consider the production of alarm clocks, toys and bedside reading.

Japanese 'music therapist' Miyashita Fumio (who passed away a couple of years ago) found yet another way to earn his living with people's sleep. He built a reputation for himself as a composer of 'Healing Music'. Studying oriental philosophy and medical science, he developed a new approach to understanding what happens in the brain during sleep, coming to the conclusion that: 'The comfortable refrain of [lengthy, monotonous] music can relax the "left brain" and unravel the "right brain" and maintain a good balance of the whole brain'. In the late 1990s and early 2000s he organised several 'inemuri (sleep) concerts' of 'healing music' during which the otherwise restless audience could find one or two hours of restful slumber. He estimated that 60,000 people had experienced 'good sleep' in the seven years of his concert series. In specialised shops there is an embarrassing choice of similar products. Kelly Howell's *Deep Stress Relief* (on two CDs), Jeffrey Thompson's *Delta Sleep System: Fall Asleep – Stay Asleep – Wake Up Rejuvenated* and Tom Kenyan's *Deep Rest* are but a few of the examples.

It therefore probably comes as no surprise that topics related to sleep and sleep research have been taken up not only by producers of exhibitions, literature and films, but also by representatives of social and cultural studies. In the Residenzgalerie Salzburg, an art exhibition (Oehring 2006) invited people to think about sleep, as did exhibitions in Dresden and London (2007–2008;

© Frank & Timme   Verlag für wissenschaftliche Literatur

Deutsches Hygiene-Museum and Wellcome Trust 2007a, b), jointly organised by the Hygiene-Museum and the Wellcome Trust in London, which combined an explanation of sleep medicine with art. Christopher and Michael Dack directed the film *Sleep* (2003) in which a person joined a sleep-deprivation study – the start of a dramatic plot. In *Sleep* (1996), made for TV by director Frank Chindamo, an innocent nap at work leads to a nightmare and in *La science des rêves* (Science of Sleep; 2006), director Michel Gondry has his main character trying to lead the girl that he is in love with into the world of his dreams. For Austrian TV, Susanne Roussow directed *Rettet den Schlaf!* in June 2006, in which reactions by Viennese on the possibility of public daytime nap facilities were tested. Andy Warhol's artistic experiment from the 1960s, *Sleep* (1963), in which he filmed John Giorno sleeping for hours, suddenly evokes new interest. Literature is equally prolific, dealing with both scientific and social aspects of sleep and sleep deprivation. A few examples are Jonathan Coe's *The House of Sleep* (1997), Annelies Verbeke's *Slaap!* (Sleep!; 2003); Yoshimoto Banana's *Shirakawa Yofune* (Asleep; 2001) and Kathrin Röggla's *Wir schlafen nicht* (We don't sleep; 2004).

After 2000, sleep also became a respectable topic for academic dissertations and other academic work: Antje Richter (2001) investigated notions of sleep in pre-Buddhist Chinese literature; Mareile Flitsch (2004) looked at Chinese sleep culture as well, but concentrated on the heated family bed in Manjuria. Steger (2004) studied the organisation of sleep in everyday Japanese life, past and present; Kaji Megumi (cf. 2008) conducted a survey on the little things Japanese have around their beds, and Diana Addis Tahhan (cf. 2007) is currently finishing her dissertation at the University of New South Wales on co-sleeping in Japan. Smaller studies on sleep have emerged from researchers' main research projects, such as Birgit Griesecke's (2005) article on how Japanese novels experiment with sleep or William LaFleur's (2002) approach to sleep in Japan from the perspective of time use and ethics.

While the studies of sleep carried out in foreign countries have often been provoked by the observation that certain basic assumptions which researchers have related to common everyday (or every-night) occurrences such as sleep are not shared by people in the country under study, sociologists have also investigated sleep at home. Under the supervision of Sara Arber at the University of Surrey, UK, and with financial support by the EU, a group of PhD students is studying how gender and family-life influences the quality of sleep

(Hislop 2004; and currently Susan Venn and Emanuela Bianchera, in this volume, among others).

The history of sleep, whether in life or literature, has also received attention recently. Following from Marcus Noll (1994), who studied notions of sleep in Shakespeare's dramas and Georg Wöhrle (1995) who analysed what Aristotle and his contemporaries thought about hypnos, Gabriele Klug (2007, this volume) investigated German medieval literature. A. Roger Ekirch's (2001; 2005) theory that early modern British people (and beyond) generally had a biphasic sleep rhythm, divided into first and second sleep, has become widely accepted. He convincingly shows that it was common for people to wake up in the middle of the night for all kinds of activities, but at least from the perspective of German literature (Klug, personal communication) it is questionable that 'first' and 'second' sleep in fact expressed a notion of biphasic sleep. As Eluned Summers-Bremner (2008) elaborates in her cultural history of insomnia, people did not seem to have clear models of ideal sleep, and although they sometimes found it difficult to get a peaceful slumber, because they missed their lover or were disturbed by fears or bedbugs, sleep was hardly medicalised and thought of much.

The emergence of this type of medicalisation is at the centre of the dissertations by Sonja Kinzler (2005), Kenton Kroker (2007) and Matthew Wolf-Meyer (2007). While Kinzler concentrates on the process of medicalisation in connection with the emergence of the bourgoisie, Kroker sketches 2,500 years of the history of sleep and provides a detailed account of the development of sleep research in the 1960s and 1970s. As an anthropologist, Wolf-Meyer looks at doctor-patient relations, the role of the US National Sleep Foundation and the discussion on postponing the start of the school day set off by medical research results indicating that children are unable to concentrate before 9 a.m.. Simon Williams at Warwick University is guided by similar research interests. As a very prolific writer he has investigated sleep as part of medical sociology. He has also published the first monograph summarising theoretical approaches to the sociology of sleep (2005; also e.g. 2002, 2007). The recent discourse on daytime 'drowsiness' and napping at the workplace in the US has stirred the academic interest of Steve Kroll-Smith (2001, 2002; Baxter and Kroll-Smith 2005). Birgit Emich (2003) discusses sleep as part of the history of German bureaucracy and social control; and in her master's thesis, Christina Dorn (2003) discusses whether or not sleep is affected by cultural change.

Most of the researchers in the social and cultural sciences have found their way to sleep independently; they often appear unaware of the activities going on in other disciplines and other countries.

Nonetheless, cooperation is also increasing. Workshops, symposia and seminar series have been organised in a number of places and from a variety of disciplines and traditions. During the seventh biannual conference of the European Association of Social Anthropology in September 2002, Burkhard Schnepel organised a panel entitled: 'When Darkness Comes. Towards an Anthropology of the Night' (Schnepel and Ben-Ari 2005), in which he combined his own research on dreams with other papers on night and sleep. At the 2007 conference of the American Anthropology Association in Washington, D.C., medical anthropologist Doug Henry set up a panel on sleep (cf. Henry et al. 2008), most certainly the first on the topic in the history of 106 AAA meetings. In 2004, 2005 and 2006 Arber and Williams organised seminar series with sleep researchers from all over the (Western) world.

Probably the oldest interdisciplinary group discussing issues pertaining to social and cultural aspects of sleep, however, was founded in Japan by anthropologist Yoshida Shūji with the financial and organisational support of the company Lofty, a pillow producer. Since Yoshida's death the group has been led by Africa anthropologist Shigeta Masayoshi at Kyoto University in close cooperation with Kaji Megumi, vice-director of the Research Institute for Sleep and Society (RISS), which is run by Lofty. The group has organised symposia and conducted research on the sleeping place, dreams, night wear as well as the small things that people keep around their beds or futons in order to enable a sound sleep (Yoshida 2001; Suimin bunka kenkyūjo 2005). In April 2008 the group published the first university textbook on 'the culture of sleep' (Takada, Horii and Shigeta 2008). Kaji presented the results of their study on 'knick knacks' for sleep at the New Directions workshop. A remarkable result of their research is that many people keep a mobile phone next to their bed, which gives them the necessary assurance to be able to sleep (Kaji and Shigeta 2007; see also Venn and Arber's contribution in this volume).

In India, the mobile phone perhaps has magical powers too, which puts it in the world of the spirits and gods during sleep. In her poem *ghumantu telifon,* the Hindi poet Anamika gives the mobile phone a voice of its own, expressing thoughts about its life and the life of its owner:

Even when he goes to sleep
he puts me under his pillow.
While listening to the tick-tick-tick
of his watch
in my entrails
I quietly assemble texts
for him.
During the night they come from all around
all night long these silent messages
– dreams and memories –
alight like cat's eyes in the dark.

(Anamika 2005: 32; translated by Lodewijk Brunt)

Lofty in Tokyo has also developed a doll, Yumel, that can be trained to talk to people before they go to sleep; supposedly this enhances their dreams. The Japanese group has always involved sleep researchers from the fields of the natural sciences and medicine, and Japanese researchers in general are more aware of the influence of the social environment on sleep. In Europe and the US, such co-operation is less common. Yet, on 13 September 2006 Steger and Brunt were invited by the president of the World Federation of Sleep Research and Sleep Medicine Societies, David Dinges, and the president of the European Sleep Research Societies, Thomas Pollmächer, to organise a social and cultural symposium at the European Sleep Research Congress in Innsbruck; is this a signal that the sciences have realised the relevance of social and cultural factors for sleep?

New Directions

For our workshop, 'New Directions in the Social and Cultural Study of Sleep' we tried to attract people who had conducted extended case studies. Rather than a homogeneous group following the same methodology and theoretical approach, we were hoping for original approaches, questions and research methods; and we were fortunate that this was the case. Although we still cannot but help observe a 'diecentrism' (Brunt 1996: 70–85) in the social sciences and humanities and have not yet fully developed a 'nocturnal literacy' (Summers-

Bremner 2008: 8), we are gradually acquiring the methodologies and vocabulary necessary to explore new grounds. We have raised not only new intriguing questions, but have been able to find unexpected answers and connections. They point to new directions and meanings of sleep beyond the often one-sided assumptions underlying medical sleep research.

The anthropologists, sociologists, historians, scholars of literature and medical sleep researchers have spent time in archives, refugee camps, streets and bedrooms in Japan, the Netherlands, USA, India, Italy, United Kingdom, Thailand, Austria and Germany. They have conducted standardised questionnaires, interviews, participant observation and fastened actigraphs around people's wrists; they have analysed preaching, pictures, epics and questionnaires. This book is a significant product resulting from the workshop. It does not provide a comprehensive overview of the new field of what we might term 'dormatology', but we believe that we have included some exciting chapters, which offer fresh new insights into a rapidly growing field.

The book starts with three chapters (Klug, Cox, Montijn) that deal with sleep in European and North American history or historical literature, respectively. They illustrate thoughts and concerns of earlier generations and provide insight into the assumptions of modern sleep medicine. Today, Americans speak easily of the problems of sleep, of deficits and disorders, of psychological and somatic disturbance, writes Cox, arguing that people in eighteenth-century New England had a much more complex view of sleep. Sleep was considered to be punishment and an ordeal, among other matters – and this is also mentioned by Klug in her contribution on German literature from the Middle Ages.

The next three chapters are closer to the research interests of natural science and medicine, by asking what disturbs people's sleep? They explore Austrian couples (Kloesch and Dittami), British parents and their teenage children (Venn and Arber) as well as Italian women who have caregiving obligations (Bianchera and Arber). They derive from the assumption that there is something resembling an ideal sleep – a good night sleep is an uninterrupted night-time sleep – but they go further: They leave the sleep labs and look at the social environment and the overall logic of the sleepers' social situation. The last chapters have an entirely different approach when investigating how – in different places in the world – people have different ways to switch from their waking day to sleep mode (Brunt, Ben-Ari, Vogler) or out of it (Steger). Routines and material objects around the bed ensure a restful slumber and deal with the vulnerability of the sleeper – a topic that is also central to Klug's paper – along with the threat sleep poses to the fulfilment of social obligations.

Whereas for some, sleep has been the central concern of their investigation, others have come across sleep as one of the important aspects of people's life when they investigate interior design (Montijn), eighteenth-century religious thought (Cox), childhood and socialisation (Ben-Ari), city life (Brunt) or refugees (Vogler). Vogler, in particular, finds the study of sleep not only fascinating in its own right, but a helpful research tool to investigate the much more sensitive issues of threats and fears among young refugees.

Each chapter in this book tells its own story and can be read separately, but in many instances the different stories speak to each other, emphasising certain arguments made by others or adding a new perspective. Despite the different approaches, there are recurrent issues discussed throughout the book.

Status Differentials

Where one sleeps, under what circumstances, with whom, how long and how well are all matters of degree, determined by gender, age, class, race, income, educational level and other differences in status. Kloesch and Dittami, Venn and Arber, Bianchera and Arber, Klug, Steger, Vogler and Brunt all show that sleep can be very different for men and women – even if they sleep together. We all have heard about men snoring and keeping women awake, but the differences are more complex. Kloesch and his colleagues have found that Austrian women's sleep is more disrupted when they sleep with their partner than alone, whereas for men it is the other way round. At this point they are still left speculating about the reasons. It is interesting that German-language literature of the Middle Ages (Klug in this volume) ascribed alertness during the night and protection to women's roles. The brave knight protects the lady of his heart against giants and dragons during the day, but he in turn is taken care of by the young maiden while he puts his head to rest after long exhausting journeys.

Nowadays, women have to be alert and occasionally get up at night because of their caring roles for children or other members of the family living under the same roof. In Germany the word *Ammenschlaf* is used for the very light sleep of wet nurses or young mothers. Values of masculinity sometimes dictate that men get up early to display the control they have over their bodies, but

18

Steger shows that in many cases women get up even earlier to help the menfolk to get up on time and support their transition to the performance of social duties.

Age is another quality that changes our status in human societies. Bianchera and Arber, Venn and Arber as well as Ben-Ari point out several phases in the lives of women and/or children that have far-reaching consequences for their sleeping behaviour. Women start out as babies and toddlers and develop into girls, young women, married women, mothers and grandmothers; in the course of these phases, accentuated by *rites de passage* they experience more or less dramatic changes in their sleeping responsibilities and sleeping conduct. From Bianchera and Arber's contribution it is clear that in Italy, where extended families are living under one roof and the public welfare system is not very well developed, these phases are perhaps more pronounced than elsewhere in Western Europe.

Closely connected with age is the 'family cycle'. The young, romantic couple has sleeping arrangements that differ notably from the family with young children and the elderly couple whose children have moved to their own houses. Ben-Ari elaborates the routines small children in middle class families develop at bedtime: story telling, undressing, washing, brushing teeth and tucking under the blanket. The 'key cultural scenario' as well as the exact timing is negotiated between children and carers. And it is interesting to realise the differences in the assumptions that surround the issue. Bedtime is among the things that Austrian children, for example, have only little input in deciding, whereas Japanese children are given much more autonomy on the issue (cf. Steger 2004: 374–400). Contrary to many households in India, where entire families sleep together in a single room, middle class families in Western societies usually arrange for a rigid division of the house in separate bedrooms for parents and children and for boys and girls. The familial hierarchy and power relations in every society determine who has the power to wake the others and how to avoid waking those who want to sleep.

Social class in the broadest sense of the term makes for completely different worlds within societies. In her study of several centuries of bed culture in the Netherlands, Montijn shows how much money people were (and still are) willing to spend on their beds in order to improve their social reputation. She mentions bedding material so expensive that people actually sleep elsewhere so as to avoid spoiling these goods. Only people with big houses and service personnel were able to sufficiently air the beds in order to get rid of bedbugs: a plague with which innumerable generations of people must have struggled. By means of social housing, authorities including social reformers and hygienists have – often successfully – attempted to influence the lower classes' sleeping habits and bedroom arrangements, but people have been equally persistent in resisting some of the ideas. Social class influences sleep habits in India as well. Poor people often have to sleep on the pavement, cuddled together as a family or on their rickshaw to protect their few belongings.

Morals, Rules and Regulations

Different norms and values attached to sleep lead to different conceptions about the way we have to deal with sleep and sleeping behaviour: the place where to sleep and the circumstances, but of course also the time and schedule. Steger elaborates on Japanese values with regard to early rising and shows how they have been an integral part of organised nationalist movements. A responsible person should show control over his or her desires; an acceptable manner to show this is by sacrificing sleep and especially by getting up early regardless of the length of sleep. Similar notions are also to be found in the contributions by Brunt, Klug and Montijn. Would early rising be a universal demand? It certainly can be found in the teachings of all the religions and quasi-religious ideologies that had their origins in Asia: Sickism, Jainism, Hinduism, Buddhism, Confucianism, Judaism, Christianity and Islam. Especially in monasteries, early-morning prayers or meditation are a crucial part of daily routine, and lay people are included in similar routines. The muezzin wakes up the entire neighbourhood – believer or not – before daybreak. The first thing for a yogi to reach *nirvana* is to be frugal in all things, especially sleeping. He must not sleep too much and has to get up early! These examples show that the main reason for demanding early rising is for people to learn self-discipline and devotion as well as integrate their bodies with social obligations.

This is also obvious in institutions such as prisons and hospitals or shelters for the homeless where early rising is an important part of the general regime and an important device to depersonalise the inhabitants and rob them of their individuality. In studies about the homeless there are ample references to early rising (cf. also Rensen 2003). Liebow (1993: 28) points out an important hardship of shelter life for women in Washington, D.C.. They have to get up at 5.30 a.m. and be out of the shelter by 7.00 a.m. 'It was not simply the fact of having to get up and out, but rather that the women had to do this every day of the week, every day of the year', says Liebow, 'no matter what the weather or how they felt [...] The occasional opportunity to stay in bed an extra hour or two was desperately missed, [...] not being able to sleep in, ever, especially on a weekend, was seen by many as a major deprivation that unfairly set them apart from the rest of the world'.

But the rest of the world has to adjust their bodies and integrate into society as well. Social status is expressed by the hour one has to wake up. Factory workers start earlier than office employees. In some modern institutions such as small companies that employ creative and artistic staff, rigid schemes are frowned upon. Creative people don't need others to stimulate them to go to sleep or wake up; they are fully capable of deciding for themselves. They are task and deadline oriented, and can thus be allowed some flexibility in how they arrange their work.

To the degree that medical doctors express their feeling that people should go to sleep at fixed hours in order to be able to get up early after a sufficient period of sleep (preferably: eight hours), they might be considered as *moral entrepreneurs* – agencies who try to develop the morals and reasoning that guide and justify our behaviour. Bedtime rituals and the sleeping environment, that is, sleep hygiene, are based on scientific grounds and are also very much 'embedded' within sleep educators' belief systems.

Co-sleeping

Morals and rules concerning the question of who you are allowed to sleep with are quite elaborate as well. In the Netherlands, boys and girls may sleep in one room as long as they are completely 'innocent' of gender differences; but parents normally start keeping them apart very early and preferably even provide babies with a room of their own. There is greater tolerance towards girls or women sleeping together than towards boys or men. But for people who are used to sleeping in their own bedroom from early childhood onwards, it can be rather difficult to sleep with any strangers around – men or women – unless of course the context would be sexual. Yet in Dutch hospitals, for instance, patients share bedrooms with members of both sexes. Would that be because sick people are not supposed to have an identity that is sexual?

In the US not only sleep research, but also popularising of the related knowledge is probably the most advanced. One of the teachings concerns bedtime; children, as Ben-Ari elaborates, are supposed to become independent by sleeping in their own room from an early age onwards. If possible, the sleeping room, and especially the bed, should not be used for and (thereby) be connected with daytime activities in order to facilitate a sound, uninterrupted sleep. It is thus most striking that even today, universities build dormitories with shared rooms for their undergraduates, regardless of the financial situation of the students (or their parents). The ideology behind this policy of having students share a bedroom, often with a complete stranger, after they had spent all their life sleeping alone, has yet to be properly analysed. However, as one of Steger's students at the University of Pennsylvania, Philadelphia (2004/05) found out, apart from exam stress and demands to socialise at night, the difficulty in adjusting to another person's presence and the divergence of sleep rhythms are the main disturbances of sleep. As another student discovered, these difficulties were experienced by students from a 'Western' background but not by those of South Asian origin who participated in her study.

In India co-sleeping is perfectly normal, except perhaps in some special circles. Formerly the institution of *purdah* – the rigid separation between men and women – divided the world into a strictly supervised private, female, part and the public, male, part. There are always persons moving more or less freely through the 'forbidden' space – provided they are emasculated and impotent. Examples are eunuchs, lower-class servants or young children – in short, typical *non-persons* who are vital for the smooth functioning of the special world but who are not capable of damaging the protected individuals.

Although at first glance, co-sleeping habits in other societies would indicate a casualness of 'who sleeps by whom' (Caudill and Plath 1974), upon closer investigation this is not the case. Even in the narrow and instable hut of the Karenni refugees, a room division is in place, if sometimes only symbolically with a piece of cloth (cf. Vogler, this volume). Similar rules exist in India (Shweder et al. 2003). The loss of virginity, incest and rape for women or the fear of (symbolic) castration for men, respectively, is a motive for this, which we find already in German medieval literature. On the other hand, pre-teenage children and same-sex siblings find protection and peace of mind in the presence of others they can trust, especially the mother or grandmother. The Japanese expression *kaya no soto*, being outside the mosquito net, refers to

© Frank & Timme   Verlag für wissenschaftliche Literatur

people who are outside of the community and therefore do not know what is going on, while everybody else (under the mosquito net) does.

Getting into Sleep Mode

Children and adults often have their special bedtime rituals or what Ben-Ari calls 'key cultural scenarios'; drinking a glass of wine, for instance, or reading, watching TV or listening to some music. Some people cannot go to sleep unless they have said their prayers, whilst others have to take a bath. These routines give them peace of mind and gradually put them into sleep mode.

The way people sleep is also extremely varied and little is known about it. Generally speaking there are only a few other people around when somebody is asleep. Even in crowded places sleeping tends to be considered as a private activity. In India one might be able to see people in every conceivable state while sleeping, but many sleepers in the public domain have symbolic ways to ensure at least the appearance of privacy. Sleepers take their shoes off and by putting a newspaper, shawl or towel over one's head, or turning one's back towards the crowd they demonstrate that they are 'away' for a while. In middle-class homes around the world, on the other hand, women who wear make-up remove it before going to sleep – or rather, change from their daytime make-up into their night-time make-up.

In some countries there are beds for sleeping, in other countries people sleep on some kind of mattress, right on the floor. There are different preferences – some for 'hard beds' and some for 'soft beds' – usually motivated by medical reasons. It is not exceptional to hear somebody say that it is 'bad for her back' to sleep in a soft bed, just as easily as one can hear somebody argue for the opposite point of view.

Security

Sleepers temporarily renounce their consciousness off the world. This means that the sleeper is vulnerable to a variety of threats and also that sleep potentially endangers social order. 'Sleep could be counted as a threat to the rational order, to the spiritual and civic as well, a threat to the economy, a threat to communication between the divine and mortal creation', writes Cox. One of the greatest fears was to die during sleep (see also Klug's chapter), and religious people had to prepare themselves for this eventuality every night. Even in the 1970s, boys in a catholic-school dormitory in Northern Italy were told to lie beautifully straight on their backs and cross their arms over their chests so that they would hold the opposite shoulder, and say their prayer and would thus be prepared for death during their sleep (Stefano, personal communication). Of course, the boys felt (at least in hindsight) that this sleeping position was mostly imposed to prevent them from masturbating.

Sexuality is frequently connected with sleep. Often women seem to be more frightened of this than men. Their sexual integrity is at stake and they stand up against an intruder who is likely to be physically stronger. If consensual, however, women feel that they sleep better if they have sex in the evening, even if this is only subjective, as Kloesch and Dittami found out. Moreover, as Klug's contribution shows, the fear of castration in sleep, whether actually or symbolically, is a recurrent topic for men. One solution to ward off the threat is co-sleeping with trustworthy persons, another is to retreat to a safe bedroom (cf. also Steger 2004: 359–361).

Some people find it impossible to sleep unless doors are closed. In Dutch there is a saying about the 'safety of the bedroom'. But not everyone can afford proper and stable housing. Refugees often have to live in rather permeable housing, not only because of their poverty, but also because welfare organisations sometimes do not approve of certain materials. Safety can also be threatened by the forces of war and natural disasters. Not only earthquakes and heavy storms and fire, but also attacks by animals, varying from the bedbugs already mentioned to mosquitoes, snakes and wild boars. And if one does not have housing at all, things are much worse still. Recently some people sleeping on the pavement in Mumbai were run over by a well-known Bollywood film star in the middle of the night. The explanation given to the press was that the man had been manoeuvring his car and had overlooked the group of sleepers.

In terms of vulnerability at night, not only bedrooms are locked at night, but also compounds, neighbourhoods and – in the past – even complete cities. In the Indian city of Ahmedabad, the *pol* – a group of houses belonging to the same family group, occupational group or caste – can be closed off from the outside world by gates. The same principle can be seen in the ancient inner cities of Varanasi, Surat and Jaipur. And of course in many other parts of the world. The original *getto* of Venice, however, was meant to prevent the inhabitants from roaming the streets of the city at night.

Sometimes attacks on the safety of sleep have a supernatural character. Vogler talks about the *nats* in Burma who have to be appeased. The devil and vampires are well-known examples in the West. In some circles people tried to protect themselves from these dangers by having a religious object (a cross) at hand or by surrounding themselves with garlic – supposedly effective at warding off wandering bloodsuckers.

The night is sometimes a time of horror when people who try to relax are attacked by all kinds of emotions they had suppressed during the day: loneliness, *angst*, sorrow and pain. The questions of vulnerability and safety are summarised by Klug in her historical analysis of sleep in German medieval literature: 'Today, many people can hardly imagine the various threats our medieval ancestors were exposed to in the dormant part of their lives, comfortably settled as they are in centrally heated bedrooms and safe apartments with the doors locked at night. While sleeping, they thought themselves to be surrounded by quite a number of dangers, real as well as imagined ones, some of which are still able to frighten us today while others seem quite remote from what we fear.' The common notion, if any, underlying all the sleep-related fears may be the idea of a dangerous loss of control and the inability to defend oneself in sleep.

Rituals

Such threats can be kept at bay by routines or rituals that constitute the transformation from social life to sleep. This transformation from one state to the other is marked, no matter how privately or secretively this might take place.

Kaji's contribution to the Vienna workshop considers some of these rituals. 'During the day I look after the children and have work to do', says one female informant in the research sample, 'and I have no time to relax and read books, so I just want a little peaceful time to read a book before I go to sleep'. 'So as to study as much as I can before sleeping', explains another person, why he goes to sleep with a study book. In the majority of responses, according to Kaji, the main idea in reading a book was not to understand its contents, but to provide 'a change of mood'. The same goes for listening to music and taking all kinds of objects along. A man cannot sleep without a certain jug half filled with water; a woman has to have her special towel around her neck or some small blanket.

Several informants could only sleep after they had cleaned their ears with an ear pick – a frequent childhood memory.

This is similar to the rituals people conduct in the morning after a good night's sleep. 'Coffee and the newspaper' is a standard means for many people in (not only) the Netherlands to really wake up and become 'human' again. Steger (2005 and this volume) writes about similar topics in her contribution on 'early rising'. Advocates of early rising in Japan suggest, for example, listening to music, doing yoga or gymnastics and enjoying an extended breakfast.

Sleep Civilisation

As a consequence of globalisation, local habits and values make way for global perspectives. Ben-Ari seems to assume a global bedtime ritual for children in the middle classes. In the same vein we might expect that sleep and sleeping practices slowly but securely become identical all over the world. The siesta might disappear from Spain and the rest of the Mediterranean area and countries such as Japan and India will become monophasic sleep societies. Or, to provide a different scenario, the campaign for power-naps might become so successful that all the societies of the world will change into napping cultures[1]. The development of widely different sleep cultures into a single global one might be aided by medical assumptions. These are very powerful and prestigious, and as many other medical principles have conquered the world, why wouldn't this be possible in the arena of sleep?

We are on our way. Talking of 'oversleep' expresses some sort of underlying assumptions about the right amount of time people have to sleep; the same goes for the notion that good sleep is 'uninterrupted sleep'. In the eyes of many medical doctors and health educators sleep is 'instrumental': it is meant to recuperate the body and it is meant to guarantee a happy and healthy life. But sleep can also be 'expressive': sleep for sleep's sake, sleep, perhaps as a way of life, a work of art. Wasn't this what Andy Warhol tried to express in his sleep film?

Might such a global sleep civilisation be possible? We don't think so. Better knowledge about the way people behave in different parts of the world could indeed lead to adaptation of one's own ways of doing things but can lead to

....

1   For an elaboration of sleep cultures see Steger and Brunt 2003: 15–20; Steger 2004: 107–140.

fierce opposition and loathing as well. And even if the entire world were transformed into one big middle class, it would not automatically lead to uniformity of thinking and acting. People are moved by many other conditions as well – climate, historical background, ethnicity and nationality to mention just a few. Rather than assuming that the population of the world sleeps eight hours a night and is awake the rest of the time, we should probe into the different world views so as to better understand why people think and behave the way they do. A new dormatology should clearly strive in this direction.

Bibliography

ANAMIKA (2005) *Khurduri hatheliyan*. New Delhi: Radhakrishna Prakashan.

BAXTER, VERN AND STEVE KROLL-SMITH (2005) 'Normalizing the Workplace Nap: Blurring the Boundaries between Public and Private Space and Time', *Current Sociology* 53(1): 33–55.

BEN-ARI, EYAL (2003) 'Sleep and Night-Combat in Contemporary Armed Forces. Technology, Knowledge, and the Enhancement of the Soldier's Body', BRIGITTE STEGER AND LODEWIJK BRUNT (eds) *Night-time and Sleep in Asia and the West. Exploring the Dark Side of Life*. London: RoutledgeCurzon, 108–126.

BRUNT, LODEWIJK (1996) *Stad*. Meppel and Amsterdam: Boom.

CAUDILL, WILLIAM AND DAVID W. PLATH (1974) 'Who Sleeps by Whom? Parent-Child Involvement in Urban Japanese Families', TAKIE SUGIYAMA LEBRA AND WILLIAM P. LEBRA (eds): *Japanese Culture and Behavior. Selected Readings*. Honolulu: University of Hawai'i Press, 277–312.

DHM [DEUTSCHES HYGIENE MUSEUM] DRESDEN AND WELLCOME TRUST (2007a eds) *Schlaf & Traum*. Wien et al.: Böhlau.

DHM [DEUTSCHES HYGIENE MUSEUM] DRESDEN AND WELLCOME TRUST (2007b eds) *Sleeping and Dreaming*. London: Black Dog Publishing.

DORN, CHRISTINA (2003) 'Der Schlaf: eine natürliche Konstante im kulturellen Wandel?' (summary of MA thesis), *Volkskunde in Rheinland-Pfalz: Jahresbericht* 18(1): 26–32.

EKIRCH, A. ROGER (2001) 'Sleep We Have Lost. Pre-Industrial Slumber in the British Isles', *The American Historical Review* 106(2): 343–385.

EKIRCH, A. ROGER (2005) *At Day's Close. Night in Times Past*. New York: W. W. Norton.

EMICH, BIRGIT (2003) 'Zwischen Disziplinierung und Distinktion: Der Schlaf in der frühen Neuzeit', *Werkstatt Geschichte* 34: 53–75.

FLITSCH, MAREILE (2004) *Der Kang. Eine Studie zur materiellen Alltagskultur bäuerlicher Gehöfte in der Manjurei*. Wiesbaden: Harrassowitz (= Opera Sinologica 14).

GRIESECKE, BIRGIT (2005) 'Intime Experimente: Unterwegs in japanischen Schlaflaboren mit Ariyoshi, Tanizaki und Kawabata', *Nachrichten der Ostasiatischen Gesellschaft (NOAG)* 177/178: 7–36.

HAYAISHI OSAMU (2004) 'Recent Progress in Sleep Research. Biological, Clinical and Social Impact', *Sleep and Biological Rhythms* 2(1): 2.

HENRY, DOUG, DANA MCCLELLEN, LEON ROSENTHAL, DAVID DEDRICK AND MELISSA GOSDIN (2008) 'Is Sleep Really for Sissies? Understanding the Role of Work in Insomnia in the U.S.', *Social Science and Medicine* 66(3): 715–726.

HIBBERT, KATHARINE (2007) 'Ways to Make You Think Better', *The Guardian* 8 November: 7–9.

HISLOP, JENNY (2004) *The Social Context of Women's Sleep: Perceptions and Experiences of Women Aged 40 and Over*. Unpubl. PhD thesis. University of Surrey.

KAJI MEGUMI (2008) 'Isogashi bijinesupāson koso "nemuri" ni tsuite kangaete hoshii' (I would like to make the busy business person think about sleep), *Nikkei Business online* 1 April, http://business.nikkeibp.article/nba/20080326/151317.

KINZLER, SONJA (2005) *Das Joch des Schlafs. Die wissenschaftliche Problematisierung von Schlaf und Schlaflosigkeit im bürgerlichen Zeitalter*. Unpubl. PhD thesis. International University Bremen.

KLUG, GABRIELE (2007) *'Wol ûf, wir sullen slâfen gan!' Der Schlaf als Alltagserfahrung in der deutschsprachigen Dichtung des Hochmittelalters*. Frankfurt et al.: Peter Lang.

KROLL-SMITH, STEVE (2000) 'The Social Production of the "Drowsy Person"', *Perspectives on Social Problems* 12: 89–109.

KROLL-SMITH, STEVE (2003) 'Popular Media and Excessive Daytime Sleepiness. A Study of Rhetorical Authority in Medical Sociology', *Sociology of Health and Illness* 25(6): 625–643.

KROKER, KENTON (2007) *The Sleep of Others and the Transformation of Sleep Research*. Toronto: University of Toronto Press.

LAFLEUR, WILLIAM (2002) 'Adjusting the Body Clock: Archaic Aspirations and Contemporary Chemicals', WALTER SCHWEIDLER (ed.): *Zeit: Anfang und Ende / Time: Beginning and End. Ergebnisse und Beiträge des Internationalen Symposiums der Hermann und Marianne Straniak Stiftung Weingarten 2002*. St. Augustin: Academia Verlag, 417–430.

LIEBOW, ELLIOT (1993) *Tell Them Who I Am. The Lives of Homeless Women*. New York: Penguin.

MELBIN, MURRAY (1987) *Night as Frontier*. New York: The Free Press.

MOALLEM, JON (2007) 'The Sleep-Industrial Complex', *The New York Times* 18 November. http://www.nytimes.com/2007/11/18/magazine.

NOLL, MARCUS (1994) *An Anatomy of Sleep. Die Schlafbildlichkeit in den Dramen William Shakespeares*. Würzburg: Königshausen & Neumann (= Kieler Beiträge zur Anglistik und Amerikanistik 8).

OEHRING, ERIKA (2006 ed) *Süßer Schlummer: Der Schlaf in der Kunst*. Berlin and München: Deutscher Kunstverlag.

RENSEN, PETER (2003) 'Sleep Without a Home. The Embedment of Sleep in the Lives of the Rough Sleeping Homeless in Amsterdam", BRIGITTE STEGER AND LODEWIJK BRUNT (eds) *Night-time and Sleep in Asia and the West. Exploring the Dark Side of Life.* London: RoutledgeCurzon, 87–107.

RICHTER, ANTJE (2001) *Das Bild des Schlafes in der altchinesischen Literatur.* Hamburg: Hamburger Sinologische Gesellschaft (= Hamburger Sinologische Schriften 4).

RICHTER, ANTJE (2003) 'Sleeping Time in Early Chinese Literature', BRIGITTE STEGER AND LODEWIJK BRUNT (eds) *Night-time and Sleep in Asia and the West. Exploring the Dark Side of Life.* London: RoutledgeCurzon, 24–44.

RÖGGLA, KATHRIN (2004) *Wir schlafen nicht.* Frankfurt am Main: Fischer.

SCHNEPEL, BURKHARD AND EYAL BEN-ARI (2005 eds) *When Darkness Comes ... Towards an Anthropology of the Night = Paideuma 51.*

SCHWARTZ, BARRY (1973) 'Notes on the Sociology of Sleep', ARNOLD BIRENBAUM AND EDWARD SANGRIN (eds) *People in Places. The Sociology of the Familiar.* London: Nelson, 18–34.

SHWEDER, RICHARD A. WITH LENE BALLE-JENSEN AND WILLIAM GOLDSTEIN (2003) 'Who Sleeps by Whom Revisited', RICHARD SHWEDER: *Why Do Men Barbecue? Recipies for Cultural Psychology.* Cambridge, MA and London: Harvard University Press, 46–73.

STEGER, BRIGITTE (2003) 'Getting *Away* with Sleep: Social and Cultural Aspects of Dozing in Parliament', *Social Science Japan Journal* 6(2): 181–197.

STEGER, BRIGITTE (2004) *(Keine) Zeit zum Schlafen? Kulturhistorische und sozialanthropologische Erkundungen japanischer Schlafgewohnheiten* ((No) time to sleep? – Cultural history and social anthropology of Japanese sleep habits). Münster: LIT.

STEGER, BRIGITTE (2005) 'Creating Time for Enjoyment, Creating Positive Energy: Why Japan Rises Early', *Paideuma* 51: 181–192.

STEGER, BRIGITTE (2006) 'Sleeping Through Class to Success: Japanese Notions of Time and Diligence', *Time & Society* 15 (2–3): 197–294.

STEGER, BRIGITTE (2007) *Inemuri. Wie die Japaner schlafen und was wir von ihnen lernen können* (*Inemuri.* How the Japanese sleep and what we can learn from them). Reinbek: Rowohlt.

STEGER, BRIGITTE AND LODEWIJK BRUNT (2003a eds) *Night-time and Sleep in Asia and the West. Exploring the Dark Side of Life.* London: RoutledgeCurzon. (paperback: Vienna: Department of East Asian Studies, Japanese Studies Section, University of Vienna 2006).

STEGER, BRIGITTE AND LODEWIJIK BRUNT (2003b) 'Introduction: Into the Night and the World of Sleep', BRIGITTE STEGER AND LODEWIJK BRUNT (eds) *Night-time and Sleep in Asia and the West. Exploring the Dark Side of Life.* London: RoutledgeCurzon, 1–23.

SUIMIN BUNKA KENKYŪJO (2005 eds) *Netoko-jutsu* (The technique of the sleeping place). Tōkyō: Popura-sha.

SUMMERS-BREMNER, ELUNED (2008) *Insomnia: a Cultural History.* London: Reaction Books.

TAHHAN, DIANA ADIS (2007) 'Two Plus One Still Equals Two: Inclusion and Exlusion in the Japanese Family', PETER BACKHAUS (ed.) *Familienangelegenheiten*. München: iudicium (= Japanstudien 19), 151–168.

TAKADA AKIKAZU (1993) *Nemuri wa hyakuyaku no chō* (Sleep is the universal cure). Tōkyō: Kōdansha.

TAKADA MASATOSHI, HORII TADAO AND SHIGETA MASAYOSHI (2008) *Suiminbunka o manabu hito no tame ni* (For students of sleep cultures). Kyōto: Sekai Shisōsha.

VERBEKE, ANNELIES (2003) *Slaap!* (Sleep!) Breda: De Geus.

WILLIAMS, SIMON J. (2002) 'Sleep and Health. Sociological Reflections on the Dormant Society', *Health: An Interdisciplinary Journal for the Social Study of Health, Illness and Medicine* 6(2): 173–200.

WILLIAMS, SIMON J. (2005) *Sleep and Society: Sociological Ventures Into the (Un)known*. London: Routledge.

WILLIAMS, SIMON J. (2007) 'The Social Etiquette of Sleep: Some Sociological Reflections and Observations', *Sociology* 41(2): 313–328.

WITTMER-BUTSCH, ELISABETH MARIA (1990) *Zur Bedeutung von Schlaf und Traum im Mittelalter*. Krems: Medium Aevum Quotidianum.

WÖHRLE, GEORG (1995) *Hypnos, der Allbezwinger. Eine Studie zum literarischen Bild des Schlafes in der griechischen Antike*. Stuttgart: Steiner.

WOLF-MEYER, MATTHEW (2007) *Urban Nocturne: Sleep Medicine, Governmentality, and the Production of 'Everyday Life'*. Unpubl. PhD thesis. University of Minnesota Twin Cities.

YOSHIDA SHŪJI (2001 ed.) *Suimin bunka-ron (Essays on Sleep Culture)*. Tōkyō: Heibonsha.

YOSHIMOTO BANANA (2001) *Asleep*. transl. by Michael Emmerich. Canongate: Grove Press.

Dangerous Doze: Sleep and Vulnerability in Medieval German Literature

GABRIELE KLUG

> ,pfî, ir zagen boese,'
> sprach der helt guot,
> ,wolt ir slâfende
> uns ermordet hân?
> daz ist sô guoten helden
> noch vil selten her getân.'
> (Nibelungenlied, *Stanza 1847*; de Boor 2003: 564)

> (*'Fie, you evil cowards,' said the valiant hero,*
> *'did you want to murder us in our sleep tonight?*
> *Such a fate was surely never intended for brave warriors like us.'*) [1]

Introduction

In recent years, the 'dormant third of our lives' has attracted increasing academic interest in the social and cultural sciences. We have become aware of the importance of sleep and have begun to understand what a multi-faceted and complex phenomenon 'death's brother' is. The role that sleep played in past epochs and the way in which it was represented in the literature of those times, however, remains largely unexplored. Based on the assumption that finding out more about what our ancestors thought about sleep will enhance our understanding of our own contemporary culture of sleep, I have started to explore the culture of sleep in the Middle Ages and thoroughly analysed German literature written between approximately 1150 and 1350 AD (cf. Klug 2007). The German literature of that epoch may be roughly divided into the epic and the lyric genre (there had been no plays written by this time) accord-

---

[1] All English translations of original passages from Middle High German texts were made by the author herself.

ing to formal aspects, and into secular and religious texts according to thematic aspects. The best-known texts belong to the epic genre, comprising heroic epics such as the *Nibelungenlied* (De Boor 2003) and Arthurian epics such as *Parzival* or *Tristan und Isolde* (Spiewok and Buschinger 1992). The most important text type of the lyric genre is certainly the courtly love poetry known as *'Minnesang'*. Sleep plays a role in all of these text types. Indeed, the universal presence of sleep in literature is the first thing that strikes the scholar of literature. To expatiate on all aspects of sleep as a cultural concept and a literary motif in the Middle Ages – even if it is only German culture that is analysed – would go far beyond the scope of a single chapter, and I will concentrate on one specific aspect only: the dangerous potential of sleep and the vulnerability caused by it.

Vulnerability in sleep is a highly interesting and much varied subject in its own right in medieval German literature. We may well speak of a literary concept since we are dealing with quite a fixed set of culturally determined ideas that is functionalised, discussed and reshaped in poetic texts. I will use both the expressions 'vulnerability in sleep' and 'vulnerability caused by sleep', always meaning vulnerability of a sleeper, of course, though the state of defencelessness or endangerment is often not restricted to the mere stretch of time in which a person is actually asleep, but may continue in wakefulness or have lasting consequences on the person's life. This chapter elaborates on the different ways in which vulnerability occurs in the literature, and which special sleep-related fears and dangers there are. It will show how vulnerability in sleep serves various poetic functions within the texts. By dealing with the various problems related to precarious sleeping situations, the literary texts are gaining both in liveliness and in psychological depth. But literary texts are also precious keys to the cultures of historical epochs, which is why we may attempt to access sleep via texts. We must not, however, expect works of fiction to give minute accounts of reality, but they use reality as a frame of reference which they modify by using specific literary means like idealisation, contrast, irony, and many others.

Cultural Parameters

In the Middle Ages, people's thoughts and feelings about sleep were deeply ambivalent. The necessity of sleep for mental and physical health was acknowledged, but the general world view was strongly determined by Christian belief and theological perspective, which is why sleep, like many other parts of human life, was subjected to a host of both judgement and prejudice originating from the Christian tradition and supported by the holy scriptures and the authority of the fathers of the church, such as Saint Augustine (354–430 AD). According to medieval theology, the need to sleep was a divine punishment for the fall of man and a daily reminder to mankind of their sinfulness, weakness and imperfection. Therefore, sleep was seen in a rather negative light, representing ideas of remoteness from God, lost time (both in a spiritual and an economic sense), loss of control over body and soul, and absence of rational regulation. Among laymen, too, sleep was considered problematic because of its subversive quality and its supposed contradiction to the idea of an active and productive social life (cf. Hergemöller 2002: 35–36).

In the High Middle Ages, sleep was beginning to occur as a motif in its own right in German literature. Many different aspects of sleep as an everyday human experience and the whole spectrum of ideas and values connected with it become topical. This development runs parallel to a rising literary interest in other remnants of everyday culture such as housing, food and clothing and is due to the tendency of literature to 'come down to earth'. There are now texts which dwell on the question of whether it is justifiable for a lady to withdraw her favour from the knight who oversleeps an appointment with her (cf. Reinitzer 2000). Other texts discuss how eminent people such as saints or worldly rulers (one example would be emperor Charles the Great) deprived themselves of sleep for the good of the community and/or the worship of god (cf. Hergemöller 2002: 27–59; Bartsch 1965). One aspect of sleep is, however, occurring particularly often in various texts: sleep-induced vulnerability. This aspect again involves in itself a wide range of further elements, both secular and spiritual in their nature. Therefore, it occurs in both religious and worldly literature, and it is formed and reformed in many different ways.

Vulnerability in Sleep

Today, many people can hardly imagine the various threats our medieval ancestors were exposed to in the dormant part of their lives, comfortably settled as we are in centrally heated bedrooms and our safe apartments with the doors locked at night. While sleeping, they thought themselves to be surrounded by quite a number of dangers, some of which are still able to frighten us today while others seem quite remote from what we fear. Belonging to the more 'real-life' sort of dangers were surely fire, flood, physical attacks by animals or by humans (in the course of war, feud or raids), and burglary, while more transcendental threats would be evil spirits or even the devil himself trying to harm the sleeper (not solely, but often particularly via dreams). The common notion underlying all the sleep-related fears is the idea of a dangerous loss of control and the inability to defend oneself in sleep.

When medieval authors started to process these fears and threats in literary texts, they soon added other, more symbolic dimensions to them. Not only did they tell their audience of bold physical attacks on sleepers, but they also used a person's vulnerability in sleep as a metaphor for more abstract problems. The modern interpreter of medieval literature is able to recognise different types of dangers for sleepers, which were obviously always more or less present in the minds of medieval authors and their audience. I have categorised these threats, but there will always remain a certain fuzziness about such categories, as there is of course some interference between different dangers. A social component, for example, is inherent in almost all the dangers humans are facing – with the possible exception of natural catastrophes such as asteroids crashing down – since they are related in some way or the other to human interaction. My category of 'social' danger means that it is most threatening to an individual's social life as opposed to, for example, 'spiritual' danger in other contexts, threatening his or her spiritual life, endangering his or her soul, and not denying other aspects being inherent as well.

Sleep as an Existential or Physical Danger

Medieval life was abundant with all sorts of real physical dangers to human life, as listed above. Generally, the danger of being physically attacked and being killed was constantly present as the individual's threshold of violence must be assumed to have been relatively low. In addition to these 'man-made' threats, there were dangers of a more 'natural' sort. We have historical records of many great fires and floods said to have destroyed whole town districts or even whole towns in a short time. Somebody who was fast asleep was unlikely to react fast enough to such dangers – he or she would, for example, not smell the smoke early enough to escape from the burning house. As wood was the

© Frank & Timme   Verlag für wissenschaftliche Literatur

dominant building material and houses stood very densely together, there was a great likelihood of fires, especially at night, when fireplaces were left unattended. In order to minimise this danger, night watchmen used to patrol the streets (cf. Wittmer-Butsch 1990: 28). Curiously, such dangers play no role at all in literature; there is no single literary text that tells of someone killed by fire while sleeping.

In literature, the main threat to sleep occurs if the hero's choice of time and place for sleeping is ill fated. Generally, in the Middle Ages, the 'right' time was considered to be at night, while the 'right' place was at home or some other place that provided some shelter and comfort (cf. Klug 2007: 31–33, 119–143). Choosing the wrong time and place for sleep often causes situations of existential danger for the characters, which led to their being nearly or actually killed in sleep, thus boldly underlining the notion of dangerous sleep. A fictional hero may in his sleep either be threatened by a human enemy, by a superhuman being like a giant or witch or by a beast such as a dragon. A quite dramatic example for this can be found in the heroic epic *Ortnit* (cf. Amelung and Jänicke 1871), which was written in the first half of the thirteenth century. The homonymous hero of the story rides out in search of an evil dragon devastating his land. After he has been riding for a very long time, searching in vain for the dragon, he becomes very exhausted and tired. So, he is forced to lie down in the woods to sleep – alone and unguarded. As soon as he is fast asleep, the dragon comes along. Ortnit, however, cannot hear him and does not awaken to defend himself, which is why the dragon is able to devour him right on the spot (cf. Amelung and Jänicke 1871: 74). That is the shocking end of the story – the most drastic instance of a 'vulnerated' sleeper in the older German literature. In the most popular medieval German heroic epic, the *Nibelungenlied*, the case is somewhat different. The literary characters are aware of their sleep-induced vulnerability, and they know exactly which sort of danger they are facing. The king of the Burgundians and his fellowmen had once conspired in the murder of dragon slayer and warrior Siegfried. After his death, his widow Kriemhild married king Etzel. Years later, she is still thirsting for revenge for Siegfried's death, so she invites the Burgundians to her court with the intention to have them killed. The Burgundians sense the imminent danger and spend their time in apprehension of an attack at night, with guards keeping watch while the rest are sleeping. Their awareness of their vulnerability and their precautions save their lives for the time being, and Kriemhild's warriors have to wait for another opportunity to attack (De Boor 2003: 564).

Death, however, is not the only thing literary characters have to fear during sleep – there are other sorts of bodily injury not directly causing death, such as castration for men and the loss of virginity for women, or other forms of sexual assault. Typical situations are adulterous lovers discovered by jealous husbands. In the courtly epic *Parzival*, we learn that the magician Chlinsor is castrated by the furious king of Sicily the moment he is surprised sleeping together with the queen (cf. Schirock 2003: 661). The literary description of incestuous sexual abuse can be found in a narrative called *Gregorius*. A young man has a sexual desire for his own sister. One night, he overwhelms the girl in her sleep and rapes her before she has the chance to scream. The progeny of this sinful incestuous act is the hero of this story, Gregorius, who has to cope with this hereditary flaw his whole life (cf. Hermann and Wachinger 1983). A further motif belonging to the category of physical threats is abduction or capture during sleep – something which was probably also a part of medieval reality, especially in times of feud. In some texts, we additionally encounter scenes in which small children are stolen away at night while their parents are asleep and unable to protect them (cf. Ameling and Jänicke 1871: 95).

So what becomes evident is the fact that literature is drawing from a 'reservoir' of sleep-related dangers that actually covers many (though not all) of the real-life dangers also relevant for its audience; and these dangers not only affect the body, but also what contemporaries considered to be the soul.

Sleep as a Spiritual or Metaphysical Danger

For both medieval superstition and theology the human soul was extremely vulnerable during sleep. It was threatened by evil spirits or even by the devil himself. The idea that the soul of a person sleeping by daylight could fall prey to spirits had already been common in Greek and Roman antiquity (cf. Bächtold-Stäubli 2000: vol. 6/col. 414). Additionally, medieval people were especially afraid of dying while asleep, since this would have been a sort of 'unprepared' death representing a danger to the immortal soul (the close, 'sibling-like' relationship between death and sleep was a concept going back to antiquity as well and was taken up by medieval thought). Special evening prayers and bedtime rituals (which are still sometimes practised today) were supposed to guard against any such dangerous situations or events during sleep (cf. Klug 2007; Bächtold-Stäubli 2000: vol. 6/col. 414–416).

 © Frank & Timme   Verlag für wissenschaftliche Literatur

The concept of spiritual vulnerability in sleep was further developed in literature. In medieval religious writings, sleep was always considered as a potentially sinful kind of sluggishness. Especially daytime sleep was likely to bereave people of their chance for salvation. This opinion was based on the more pragmatic message of bible passages such as Proverbs 6, 9–11: 'How long will you lie there, you sluggard? When will you get up from your sleep? A little sleep, a little slumber, a little folding of the hands to rest – and poverty will come on you like a bandit and scarcity like an armed man.' Sleep was used as a metaphor, standing for a 'sleep of the soul', remoteness from god and a dangerous entanglement in the sinful ado of worldly pleasures. The unconverted heathens were – just like the obdurate Christian sinners – compared to daytime sleepers who were not able to see the light of the sun (symbolising Christ) shine through the shutters. Their sleep was equated with a dangerous sleep of the soul – those who would not be woken up in time would have to face damnation. There was even a special genre of medieval religious literature which concentrated on this motif of the endangered sinful sleeper: the so-called 'religious alba'. The worldly alba or morning song, belonging to the literary genre of *Minnesang*, describes the situation of two secret lovers who, after having spent a night together, must not oversleep but separate at the break of day in order to avoid being discovered. In these texts, sleep is dangerous with respect to a possible disclosure of a secret and (inappropriate) sexual activity. The religious alba then converted the motif of vulnerability in sleep away from its worldly dimension into a complex spiritual meaning. In the songs, usually a guardian character ardently appeals to a nameless sleeper who represents 'the sinner' and tells him to end his obnoxious sleep before it is too late and he loses god's grace (an example of this will follow later).

In comparison to such abstract compositions, there are also more practical views on the possible threats for the souls of the sleeping. In an Austrian Benedictine monastery, an interesting text from the thirteenth century has survived which testifies to the spiritually rooted real-life fear of sleeping. This text is called the 'Seckau breviary for nuns' (Seckau being the name of the monastery where it was written) and contains rules and practical advice for the daily life in a medieval nunnery (cf. Schönbach 1876: 129–197). Detailed instructions for going to bed and sleeping safely are a vital part of its contents, as they have always been a part of the Benedictine Rule. The breviary suggests how the nuns should arrange for a spiritually safe sleep in the evening. They are advised to sprinkle the dormitory with holy water and to seal their five senses with the sign of the Holy Cross.

> *So ir iwich denne slafen legent, so sult ir besigelen ur vinf sinne mit dem heligen cruce. ê ir uch nider leget, so sol ain swestr umb gen unt daz slafhus mittem wich prunnen vil flizlichen besprengen. (Schönbach 1876: 142)*

> *(When you go to sleep, you should seal your five senses with the Holy Cross. Before you lie down in bed, one of the nuns should walk around in the dormitory and sprinkle holy water everywhere.)*

These practices, though formally Christian rituals, may be seen as magical acts and have to be considered in the context of diverse magical artefacts kept in medieval sleeping rooms (cf. Bächtold-Stäubli 2000: vol. 1/cols. 746 and 1184). The 'closing' of the five senses clearly reveals the apprehension that something obnoxious might enter a human being through the senses and via the corresponding body openings (mouth, ears, nose). In addition to these practical safety instructions, the nuns are told to do something we would probably call 'sleep hygiene' today, in so far as they should order their thoughts, i.e. remember the good things they did during the daytime and ask god to forgive them for their bad thoughts and deeds. The purpose, apart from being a preparation for sound sleep, can be seen in an indirect preparation for death. In case a nun would be 'surprised' by death in her sleep, she could hope for faster redemption provided that she had practised this clearance of conscience before going to bed. One may well label this set of advice with the term *ars dormiendi*, in reference to the well-known concept of *ars moriendi* (cf. Klug 2007: 52–58).

Sleep as a Social or Moral Danger

The third category of dangers involved in sleep has a particularly strong impact on the sleeper as a social being and his or her subjection to moral standards. In the Middle Ages, sleep as such was always on the verge of being considered a morally dubious thing (cf. e.g. Hergemöller 2002: 27). Sleeping too much or oversleeping could result in a person's loss of honour and regard. Doing one's social and economic duty as required by the ethics of one's rank in society eventually always involved more or less strict sleep control. The higher a person's social rank, the more important their control over sleep (cf. e.g. *Der Wälsche Gast*, Rückert 1965). So, somebody who slept too much, in the wrong place, at the wrong time or in the wrong situation was extremely vulnerable in a social sense and exposed to social and behavioural sanctions. By 'wrong situation', either a situation that would require some sort of action instead of sleep/passivity or a public situation is meant here. At least for people of a higher social standing, the right place to sleep had to be private and secluded from public gaze. Sanctions could range from more or less public shame and ridicule to the loss of a certain person's love or even the complete and irreversible loss of esteem.

There are quite a number of literary texts dealing with the question of how much sleep is tolerable for whom, and what may happen if one fails to control sleep. Again, it is useful to take into account that bible exegesis had a strong influence on medieval world view and consequently on medieval literature; the idea of sleep as a potential risk to a person's honour can be found in Genesis 9: 20–24. This bible passage tells the story of Noah, who drank too much wine one day and then fell asleep. In his sleep, he denuded himself. One of his sons, Ham, found him in this compromising situation and ridiculed him, while his other two sons decently looked away and covered Noah with a garment. In the biblical story, Ham is cursed and condemned for his impious behaviour and Noah is not blamed. But Noah is a holy man, and things were quite different for ordinary Christians in the Middle Ages. Even in his state of limited self awareness the sleeper was seen as responsible for the protection of his honour, symbolised not only by covering the naked body, but also by donning him- or herself with appropriate garments. This responsibility puts him in a most vulnerable moral position.

Medieval didactic literature generally preaches in favour of a strict sleep control and warns against oversleeping and the resulting loss of honour, while courtly literature in particular presents negative 'case studies'. At King Arthur's court, for example, sleep is as much subject to courtly etiquette as any other part of life. To lie down and sleep in the great hall among the courtly society of knights and ladies is considered to be extremely rude. Arthurian court ruffian Keie is the negative example – while all the other members of court pursue chivalric activities, he placidly dozes away among them, 'longing for rest instead of honour' (*ze gemache ân êre stuont sîn sin*) (Wehrli 1988: 10). Courtly etiquette actually dictates that those who would like to go to sleep have to ask the king or the lord of the castle for leave in a formal manner; thus they will not be exposed to frowns and ridicule. An example for the correct behaviour would be the young knight Parzival (cf. Schirock 2003).

One literary hero whose honour is severely damaged by sleeping in the wrong situation (though he actually did *not want* to sleep) is the young knight Kaedin in the thirteenth-century courtly epic *Tristan* written by Ulrich von Türheim (cf. Spiewok and Buschinger 1992). Kaedin is searching for amorous adventures. He soon takes to a pretty court lady and tries to persuade her to spend the night with him. The girl, whose name is Camele, fears for her virginity and refuses him, but her Lady Isolde finally orders her to comply with the young knight's wishes. Secretly, however, she gives a magical cushion to Camele and advises her to place it under Kaedin's head. As soon as that would happen, the young man would fall asleep instantly and Camele would be able to keep her virginity. The girl acts according to the advice of her Lady, and Kaedin gets an extended sleep instead of the erotic pleasure he actually sought. In the morning, when Camele takes away the cushion and Kaedin awakens from his deep sleep, he is completely disoriented and does not understand what had happened to him. He is unable to make out why he could have slept beside a beautiful girl having obviously not touched her, and he starts to seriously doubt his manliness. To make matters worse, he is ridiculed by Camele, who presents the matter as if Kaedin's quality as a lover had been a serious disappointment to her. In the end, Kaedin is the general object of ridicule for having slept instead of making love. So it can be said that magically induced sleep in this story is the means to deliberately injure a character's honour and sexual prestige, but not only that, the whole sequence can be seen as a punishment for Kaedin, who was seeking only carnal pleasure regardless of the feelings and wishes of the girl. In this respect, he stands in sharp contrast to the hero Tristan, who is a master in the art of courtly, polite love. As Kaedin is utterly failing in this art, he has to suffer symbolic castration (cf. Spiewok and Buschinger 1992: 98).

This story reveals gender-related differences concerning vulnerability in sleep. Whereas men are expected to diminish their sleep-induced vulnerability by sleep deprivation or at least sleep reduction and control, female literary characters rather tend to defend themselves by magical means, i.e. by casting sleep over their male antagonists. In fact in literature women appear to have power over sleep. Firstly they induce sleep and use sleep as a means to achieve something, and secondly they watch over men's slumber and thereby control their sleep (see below). Men seem to belong to the sphere of wakefulness and

 © Frank & Timme   Verlag für wissenschaftliche Literatur

reason while women belong to the sphere of sleep and magic. These different gender-specific ways of coping with sleep point to a dichotomy of the genders well known in Western culture and can still be traced in contemporary cultural discourses: the assumption that man stands for rationality and activity while woman stands for passivity and the irrational, dreamy sphere of life.

Specific Functionalisations of Dangerous Sleep in Literature

What are the specific textual functions the motif of vulnerability in sleep could take? As already said, dangerous sleeping was often transformed into more abstract statements by medieval authors, and at times it took the role of a special stylistic device as well. The literary functions may be text-inherent and are particularly important for the inner structure and organisation of the plot and its textual realisation. Alternatively, they may be working on the level of text impact, which means that they are mainly important for the effect a text has on its audience.

Functions on the Level of Story

Courtly chivalric literature is based on a set of specific social rules and acting directives. The principles of knighthood along with its code of honour are discussed and exemplified by this sort of literary texts of the High Middle Ages (cf. e.g. Bumke 1999: 417–430). Sleep is embedded into the system of chivalric norms like every other part of life. Particularly the way of acting towards others who are sleeping, i.e. the question of how to react properly to others' vulnerability in sleep, is dwelt on. A recurrent topic is the ritual of waking up potential combatants. Medieval knights were supposed to ride off in search of adventure in order to enhance their honour. However, daring adventure is not enough, the 'how' is an important factor as well. If a knight happens to meet another knight sleeping somewhere in the open and intends to fight him, it is his duty to wake the other before attacking him; an honourable Christian knight never would take advantage of another's vulnerability in sleep. The compliance with this rule is what makes the difference between a righteous knight and a villain, and it has to be complied with even if the other is decidedly evil and/or a super-human being. In the Middle High German epic

Rennewart, the hero Willehalm wants to defeat the evil giant Terramer, who has long been a menace to his country. When he finally finds him sleeping in the open field, he does not take advantage but wakes him up to give him the opportunity to get ready to fight. The narrator underlines Willehalm's ideal behaviour by commenting *'ein wunder ez an im was / als er in slafende vant / daz in ertotte niht sin hand'* (*'it was a wonder he did not kill him when he found him sleeping'*) (Hübner 1938: 128). In another epic called *The Younger Sigenot*, the hero Dietrich von Bern is up against a villainous giant as well, and again the warrior finds his enemy sleeping (as daytime sleeping in the open field or wood seems to be a favourite pastime of giants, which also puts an emphasis on their moral inferiority). Aloud he ponders upon the possibility of slaying the villain on the spot, and decides to wake him up:

> *Ich hân mich waerlich wol bedâht:*
> *Slueg ich dich in dem gewilde*
> *Alsô slâfend iezuo tôt,*
> *Des hett ich iemer schande.*
> *[…]*
> *Sîn degenheit im daz gebôt*
> *Daz ern nit mit der hande*
> *Wolt wecken: er gap im einen stôz*
> *Mit dem fuoze für die bruste.*
> *Dâ von erwaht der grôz. (Schoener 1928: 84)*

> (*'I pondered thoroughly upon this matter: if I slew you right here in the wilderness, fast asleep as you are, this would earn me eternal shame.'* […] *His chivalry commanded him to wake him [the giant] up, but not with his hand: with his foot he kicked the giant's breast, and thus woke him up.*)

The directive to wake up those one finds sleeping outdoors not only comprises potential male combatants, but also includes female characters – of course with a different code of acting. On one occasion Dietrich happens to find a beautiful lady sleeping in a wood. Women sleeping alone in woods or other natural sceneries are generally not common in medieval literature, but the heroic epics about Dietrich von Bern are rich in fairytale-like narrative elements, so we must not be too surprised about such a scene. For Dietrich, it is clear that he will not abuse this situation but try to wake up the lady politely and gently.

> hin vür die vrouwen er dô gie.
> er liez sich nider an ein knie.
> dô slief sî alsô vaste
> daz sî sîn dâ niht innân wart:
> sî was sô gar verslâfen.
> er sprach 'vil liebiu vrouwe zart,
> ir soltent mich niht strâfen,
> daz ich iu sus erwecket hân.'
> sî sprach 'nein, lieber herre,'
> und sach in güetlîch an. (Tuczay 1999: 75)

> (He went to the lady and kneeled down beside her. She was so fast asleep that she did not notice him: very sleepy she was. He said: 'Sweet and tender Lady, please do not reprove me for waking you up like this.' She said: 'I shall not, dear Sir', and gave him a friendly glance.)

Dietrich receives the reward for his good behaviour quite promptly, as the lady turns out to be a good fairy-like creature ready to help him.

Because it is considered to be so utterly dishonest to attack a sleeping antagonist, the mere accusation of having done so is often used as a purposeful insult. In many texts this accusation is used as a powerful provocation and seems to belong to a kind of ritualised prelude to the fight. Again it is Dietrich von Bern who is confronted with such a provocation in order to be challenged into a duel – two giants are jealous of Dietrich, because he is such a flawless knight and brave hero whose name resounds throughout the land. Therefore, they falsely accuse him of once having killed a famous giant while the latter was sleeping. They insinuate that Dietrich would never have been able to fight the giant had he been awake and ready for the attack. Dietrich in turn can do nothing other but accept the challenge – otherwise he would lose his honour in a double sense: by admitting the past shame and by shunning the fight that would punish the lie (cf. Tuczay 1999: 15).

Whereas in high medieval literature, representations of vulnerability in sleep are predominantly concerned with masculinity and male chivalric norms and values, in the prose romances of the Late Middle Ages sleep is a danger to female honour. Such a loss of female honour in sleep is the central event in the late-medieval prose romance *Sibille* (Tiemann 1977). It constitutes the pivotal event of the story, which causes all the following events to happen and sets a whole sequence of adventures in motion. Sibille, faithful wife to Charlemagne, refuses an ugly dwarf who is courting her in an indecent manner. Once the queen is sleeping alone in her chamber, unattended by her maidens, the dwarf sneaks in and watches her in her sleep. However, as soon as he starts to whisper to her of his desire, the queen wakes up and is able to successfully defend herself against the impudent dwarf. When he openly asks her to fulfil his intimate wishes right away, she gets so angry that she punches him and throws him out of her chamber. The dwarf, who is deeply offended, wants to satisfy his thirst for revenge on the queen even at the cost of his own life. Therefore he creeps into the queen's bedchamber once again and hides behind a curtain. At night, after the chamber has been closed by the valets and the queen is alone, he lies down naked beside the sleeping queen in her bed. They are found by the king like this in the morning. Interpreting what he sees as clear proof of adultery, he sentences his wife to death, but eventually spares her life and banishes her from the kingdom while the dwarf is hanged. After this, the unhappy queen has to stand the test of numerous adventures in an odyssey-like journey, before eventually being restored to happiness. The scenes in the queen's bedchamber are of vital importance in this story. It is particularly interesting to observe two things in them: Firstly, the queen is more vigilant in her daytime sleep, so she wakes up in time to prevent a possible assault, while at night she sleeps so soundly and deeply that she does not notice the dwarf at all. Secondly we learn that the queen sleeps alone at night, whereas her daytime sleep would usually have been protected by her court maidens who, however, that one day neglect their duty.

> *Als die junffrowen vernamen*
> *das ir frouwe entslaffen was*
> *da slichen sye alle vß der kammer*
> *vnd gingen vff eynen bornen*
> *das sie sich mit eynander ergetzten*
> *Sye liessen die kammer wijt vffen stene*
> *vnd nyeman bleyb dar jnn. (Tiemann 1977: 120)*

(When the maidens noticed that their lady had fallen asleep, they all sneaked out of the chamber and went to a well, where they enjoyed themselves. They left the chamber wide open, and nobody remained within.)

In literary texts of later epochs – especially in drama – servants tend not to count as full-value literary characters, which means that the main (aristocratic) characters are acting in their presence as if they were actually not there at all. In medieval literature, however, things are quite different, and particularly in the narrative of the queen Sibille, the courtly maidens – though of course they are not full plastic characters who act independently – are still characters with a specific literary function and some importance for the plot, regardless of their social status. This applies not only to the late-medieval *Sibille* narrative, but also to the courtly epic *Parzival*, which was written much earlier. When queen Herzeloyde lies asleep in her chamber, surrounded and watched over by her maidens, she is haunted by nightmares. In her sleep, she cries out and moves so violently that she nearly falls out of bed. Her maids, however, instantly come to her aid and gently wake her in order to relieve and comfort her (cf. Schirock 2003: 106).

The protection of sleep is a special motif directly linked to the concept of vulnerability in sleep, since the latter is inherent in the former. It is quite frequent and manifests itself in two different ways: On the one hand, there are numerous texts which describe scenes of physical protection of sleep, i.e. of precautions against mortal dangers (attacks). On the other hand, there are scenes in which the concept of sleep protection is transposed to a more abstract, ritual level. Curiously, it is mostly male characters who need to be protected in sleep, while female characters are often the protectors, though not always. A faithful lion, for example, watches over the sleep of the Arthurian knight Iwein (Wehrli 1988: 254). Dietrich von Bern, however, relies on a woman's protection when he sleeps. He once saved a beautiful girl from a horde of evil hunters and accompanied her on her journey afterwards. She in turn watched over his sleep and woke him when danger was imminent (we will return to this text a little later). The unlucky king Ortnit – he who is the most radical incarnation of 'vulnerability in sleep' and whose bad fate we learnt about earlier – is lacking such a human friend and protector, but he does have a dog with him. As soon as the dragon approaches the sleeping Ortnit, the dog barks to warn him, but in vain. Ortnit is not to be risen from his deep and almost comatose sleep. It is not a wholly natural sleep after all, but it symbolises a defect of character in the hero. Ortnit's deadly sleep is the peak of his progressing passivity throughout the story. Neither the most dutiful watchdog nor a human guard could have saved him. Ortnit's horrible fate serves as intertextual reference in some later epics, emphasising vulnerability in sleep as it symbolises the vulnerability of male chivalry, and pointing to the much feared notion of death in sleep.

Watching over a person's sleep is not always a matter of life or death. Apart from such practical duties of a sleep guard as chasing away insects from a sleeping person (as mentioned in a courtly narrative called *Meleranz*, cf. Bartsch 1861: 25) it often becomes a more ritualised, metaphorical kind of protection expressing exceptional love and care. Such scenes often have an almost tableau-like appearance. A lady holds the head of a sleeping knight (her husband or lover) in her lap and gently watches over his sleep, taking care that he is not disturbed by any outside influences (cf. e.g. *Moriz von Craun*, Reinitzer 2000: 65). There is one special literary genre which particularly strongly attributes the role of the guardian over male sleep to the woman: the alba. The woman has the duty of waking her lover in time before the break of day and the public attention entailed by it. The secret lovers must part, since oversleeping and being detected would be extremely dangerous for both of them. Recapitulating, it becomes evident that in most literary texts the absence or failure of the sleep guardian may have dramatic consequences for the sleeping character, and it is exactly this fact which holds great potential for literary tension. This points already to the second type of literary functions attributable to the concept of vulnerability in sleep.

Functions on the Level of Text-Audience Relationship

Let us return to Dietrich von Bern who has just saved the young girl from her persecutors. The villains are thirsting for revenge, while Dietrich and the girl are trying to escape from their sphere of power. At some point, however, Dietrich becomes exhausted (he had recently been wounded in a fight) and needs some rest. The girl promises to remain vigilant in the mean time and to wake him instantly should their persecutors come into sight. Dietrich falls into a deep sleep; after some time the villains approach. Desperately, the girl tries to wake up Dietrich, but he does not seem to hear her at all. The situation soon becomes very dangerous. She calls to Dietrich; she touches and shakes him – to no avail. Meanwhile, the persecutors with their dogs are getting nearer.

> *sî sprach 'nu wachent schiere,*
> *ald wir sîn gar verlorn.'*
> *Dô ruorte er sich daz sî ez sach.*
> *vil schiere sî zem helde sprach*
> *,ir slâfent gar ze sêre.*
> *wahent durch iuwer maneheit.'*
> *dô hôrte er niht waz sî im seit.*
> *dô ruoftes aber mêre*
> *vor zorne er ûz dem slâfe spranc*
> *und vrâgtes waz ir waere. (Tuczay 1999: 85)*

> *(She said: 'Wake up now quickly, or we shall be lost.' Then she could see him move slightly. Anon she said to the hero: 'You sleep too much. Wake up for the sake of your manliness.' But he did not hear what she said. She continued to address him, and finally, annoyed, he startled and asked her what it was.)*

There is no doubt that the villainous persecutors would have killed Dietrich in his sleep had he not woken up at the last moment. The motif of the hero's defencelessness in deep sleep, along with the narrative technique in this scene greatly enhances the suspense. It is interesting to see that the girl refers to Dietrich's 'manliness'. This should ring a bell when we remember Kaedin and Camele: again, sleep seems to contradict the concept of manliness. Whereas in the case of Kaedin it is the sexual component of manhood that's damaged when Camele symbolically castrates the hero by making him sleep, here it is the warrior aspect of manhood that's endangered by the hero's sleepiness. The female character in this text helps the hero to preserve his male prestige by chasing off sleep, while Camele deliberately damages male prestige to save her own sexual integrity. There is a precarious relationship between sleep, power, gender roles and personal identity, which serves to construct different models of action and behaviour.

There is another conclusion to be drawn at this stage. Whenever a knight falls asleep somewhere in the open nature – in a meadow, field or wood – this constitutes a crucial moment in the narrative and the development of the hero.

The otherwise strong and powerful knight is temporarily helpless. At this point various evil forces might harm him, and magical events or twists of fate might befall him without his being able to do anything against them. This creates massive tension in a text. The audience is left uncertain about the direction of the plot. In addition to Ortnit and Dietrich there are many more colourful and interesting examples of this. In the course of one of his adventures, the hero Wolfdietrich is found sleeping in the woods by a wild ugly woman. At first it seems that the woman has something evil in mind, the more so as she steals and hides his sword while he is asleep. Again the hero's state of defencelessness caused by sleep creates suspense – the audience is left in uncertainty about the true motives of the woman. She might be a friendly, harmless creature, but she might also be an evil creature (this theory would be supported by the woman's ugly outward appearance, which is usually a sign for wickedness in medieval literature). Maybe the wild woman wants to cast a spell on him or even kill him because, as we soon learn, the meadow in which Wolfdietrich is sleeping belongs to her, like all the surrounding land; so she seems to be quite a powerful creature, too. Later, however, the tension is suspended when the woman turns out to be a helpful and friendly creature. We learn that she initially mistrusted Wolfdietrich, which was the reason for her taking away his sword (cf. Amelung and Jänicke 1871: 135–137). Yet, things could well have developed in a quite different direction. Another of Wolfdietrich's adventures brings him in contact with another wild woman, but this time she is an evil creature. This woman wants Wolfdietrich to be her lover, but he refuses her. This woman, too, steals his sword, but she takes it into the woods in order to lure Wolfdietrich there. When, exhausted and tired, he finally finds her and wants his sword back, she invites him to take a little nap in her lap. He refuses – he would never consent to sleep in the lap of such a devilish creature and expose himself to her power. Now the woman gets angry and casts a spell on him – instantly Wolfdietrich falls asleep. In this magical sleep, he is utterly helpless, and the woman continues to bewitch him. Her further spells cause the hero to go mad; for half a year he has to roam the woods as a madman (cf. Amelung and Jänicke 1871: 214–215). A two-stage way of action is visible here: first, the wild woman disables Wolfdietrich by putting him to sleep. Then, using his state of defencelessness, she acts her black magic on him. With scenes like this in mind, it can be supposed that the audience of medieval texts may have been susceptible to the suspense created by precarious sleep situations.

 © Frank & Timme   Verlag für wissenschaftliche Literatur

Another important literary function of 'vulnerability in sleep' for the text-audience relationship is that of direct appeal. This function applies most of all to the religious alba. In this type of medieval lyrical poetry, sleep is equated with sin, and the sinners, who are deeply entangled in the evils and vices of the world, are compared to day sleepers who are still lying in their beds while the sun is already shining. In this metaphor, 'sleep' stands for 'not being prepared' and not being ready for the coming of the Lord. The 'sleeping' souls thus are in a state of vulnerability, because if they are surprised by the arrival of the Lord in their state of 'spiritual sleep', they cannot be redeemed and therefore lose eternal life. The speaker in these poems is in most cases a watchman-like character, who is there to awaken the sinners from their dangerous sleep. By addressing the audience directly and warning them explicitly against the threats to the soul during sleep, the watchman character achieves a particularly strong effect on the audience. This effect is still enhanced by the everyday nature of the metaphor itself. The audience is likely to know the picture he is conjuring up from their own experience: probably the majority of them have already slept in daylight, and the feeling they attribute to that experience is likely to be basically positive (though also likely to be connected with bad conscience). Now suddenly this formerly rather ordinary and positively connoted behaviour is transformed into something quite menacing by the literary text. A harmless wake-up call takes on the quality of a harsh *memento mori*. The following example may serve to illustrate this:

> *Ich wahter, ich solt wecken*
> *den sünder der dâ riuzet sêr,*
> *daz er sich tete erschrecken*
> *ûz sînes sünden schîn.*
> *[...]*
> *Nu wache ûf, sünder traege,*
> *bedenke hinder unde für,*
> *wie harte ez dir nu laege*
> *ob er dich slâfen funde*
> *Der dîn so dicke lâget*
> *und în gât durch beslozzen tür.*
> *ez wart nie sô gewâget,*
> *sît du niht weist die stunde*
> *Wann sich dîn leben endet. (Probst 1999: 81–82)*

(I, the watchman, shall wake up the sinner who lies here snoring loudly, in order to startle him away from his sinful way of life. [...] Now wake up, sluggish sinner, and think hard about how bad things would turn out for you if the one, I mean him [death], who is constantly ambushing you and who is able to come in through closed doors, would catch you sleeping. You are in great danger, since you do not know the hour when your life will end.)

Again, we notice the medieval fear of dying while asleep. The sleeper, who thinks he is safe behind locked doors, is disillusioned, and the picture of the 'sluggish' sleeper 'snoring loudly' is used in a pejorative way. We can see that the literary transformation of the late-riser motif now introduces an aspect of vulnerability into the formerly common sleep situation that is drastically new – and that is the actual art underlying this sort of appellative religious poem. This is its actual potential to startle the audience.

Conclusion

Vulnerability is an elemental aspect of sleep. German medieval literature goes much farther than just describing basic existential experiences of being exposed to real or potential dangers while sleeping. Literary texts transfer the motif of defencelessness to various psychological, spiritual and social levels. The connection between vulnerability in sleep and gender issues is of particular interest. Although women might lose their virginity during sleep, vulnerability in sleep seems to be especially related to masculinity, whereas the power over sleep may well be labelled female. So in a way, sleep in literature inverts real-life power relations – an aspect that has not been paid attention to in earlier research on sleep.

It is also fascinating to see how crucially important such a seemingly every-day experience as sleep can become for the composition of a literary text. The motif of the defenceless sleeping self exposed to various outside influences can serve different stylistic purposes in literary texts: On the level of the story, it fulfils crucial functions for plot development, plasticity of characters and the structuring of action. On the level of textual effects, it is involved in the creation of literary tension. Finally, it adds considerable depth and liveliness to the texts by helping the modern recipient reach a closer understanding not only of

© Frank & Timme   Verlag für wissenschaftliche Literatur

the cultural concepts but also of the everyday feelings and anxieties of both medieval authors and their audience.

Literature

Primary Text Sources

AMELUNG, ARTHUR AND OSKAR JÄNICKE (1871–1873 eds) *Ortnit und die Wolfdietriche nach Müllenhoffs Vorarbeiten.* 2 vols. Berlin: Weidmann.

BARTSCH, KARL (1861 ed.) *Der Pleier: Meleranz.* Stuttgart: s.n.

BARTSCH, KARL (1965 ed.) [1857] *Der Stricker: Karl der Große.* Berlin: de Gruyter.

DE BOOR, HELMUT (2003 ed.) *Das Nibelungenlied. Zweisprachig.* Köln: Parkland.

HÜBNER, ALFRED (1938 ed.) *Ulrich von Türheim: Rennewart.* Berlin: Preußische Akademie der Wissenschaften.

PAUL, HERMANN AND BURGHART WACHINGER (1984 eds) *Hartmann von Aue: Gregorius.* Tübingen: ATB.

PROBST, MARTINA (1999) *'Nû wache ûf, sünder traege.' Geistliche Tagelieder des 13. bis 16. Jahrhunderts. Analysen und Begriffsbestimmung.* Frankfurt et al.: Peter Lang.

REINITZER, HEIMO (2000 ed.) *Mauritius von Craûn.* Tübingen: Niemeyer.

RÜCKERT, HEINRICH (1965 ed.) *Der Wälsche Gast des Thomasin von Zirclaria.* Berlin: de Gruyter.

SCHIROCK, BERND (2003 ed.) AND PETER KNECHT (transl.) *Wolfram von Eschenbach: Parzival. Studienausgabe.* Berlin and New York: de Gruyter.

SCHOENER, CLEMENS (1928 ed.) *Der jüngere Sigenot, nach sämtlichen Handschriften und Drucken.* Heidelberg: C. Winter.

SCHÖNBACH, ANTON EMANUEL (1876) 'Über einige Breviarien von Sanct Lambrecht', *Zeitschrift für deutsches Altertum* 20. 129–197.

SPIEWOK, WOLFGANG AND DANIELLE BUSCHINGER (1992 eds) *Ulrich von Türheim: Tristan und Isolde. Originaltext nach der Heidelberger HS Cod. Pal. Germ. 360.* Amiens: Centre d'Études Médiévales, Université de Picardie.

TIEMANN, HERMANN (1977 ed.) *Der Roman von der Königin Sibille in drei Prosafassungen des 14. und 15. Jahrhunderts.* Hamburg: Hauswedell & Co.

TUCZAY, CHRISTA (1999 ed.) *Die Aventiurehafte Dietrichepik: Laurin und Walberan, der Jüngere Sigenot, das Eckenlied, der Wunderer.* Göppingen: Kümmerle.

WEHRLI, MAX (1988 ed.) *Hartmann von Aue: Iwein. Middle High German Text, Based on the 7th Edition by Beneke, Lachmann, Wolff.* Zürich: Manesse.

Works of Reference

BÄCHTOLD-STÄUBLI, HANNS (2000 ed.) [1927–1942] *Handwörterbuch des deutschen Aberglaubens.* 10 vols. In cooperation with Eduard Hoffmann-Krayer. Berlin: de Gruyter.

BUMKE, JOACHIM (1999) *Höfische Kultur. Literatur und Gesellschaft im hohen Mittelalter.* München: DTV.

HERGEMÖLLER, BERND-ULRICH (2002) *Schlaflose Nächte. Zur moralischen, metaphorischen und metaphysischen Bedeutung von Schlaf im Mittelalter.* Hamburg: HHL-Verlag.

KLUG, GABRIELE (2007) *'Wol ûf, wir sullen slâfen gan!' Der Schlaf als Alltagserfahrung in der deutschsprachigen Dichtung des Hochmittelalters.* Frankfurt et al.: Peter Lang.

WITTMER-BUTSCH, MARIA ELISABETH (1990) *Zur Bedeutung von Schlaf und Traum im Mittelalter.* Krems: Medium Aevum Quotidianum.

The Suburbs of Eternity:
On Visionaries and Miraculous Sleepers

ROBERT S. COX

Facing rows of sultry pews and the woollen weight of a humid afternoon, the shuffle of feet providing a restless cadence to his sermon, one might almost sympathise with Cotton Mather, the most prominent minister in colonial Boston. One can almost feel the sting of his rhetorical lash as he scolded his flock for their indifference to his efforts to save their souls, for drowsing away the precious hours in church.

> 'Is it possible!' he cried, 'What! Sleep, when you have a Blessed Saviour at Prayer in your company! The only Advocate that is to plead the Causes of Our Souls, now making the Prayer, from which the Disciples must learn how to pray for themselves; Now making the Prayer which they own Eternal Salvation depended on; And yet these Disciples fall Asleep at the Prayer!' (Mather 1719: 1)

The ire that Mather felt that day for those who turned away from the fiery word to a well-timed nap was an anger not uncommon among the clergy of the eighteenth-century English world, and perhaps particularly among Mather's black-robed brethren in New England. Sleep, for them, was a problem. Today, Americans speak easily of the problems of sleep, of deficits and disorders, of psychological and somatic disturbance, but the problem signified by Mather's ire was rather more complex. Theologians, physiologists, and philosophers, economists and moralists all wrestled with the deeper meaning of sleep, which like death (its kissing cousin) entailed a closure of the senses and a radical separation from social interaction. As the educated elite tried out physiognomy, phrenology, mesmerism, and other new technologies for plumbing the inner universe of the mind, as they tried new modes of sensing unseen relations binding the universe, sleep appeared to present an opportunity to connect the mind with the very forces that bound human and spiritual community.

Over the past decade, Brigitte Steger and Lodewijk Brunt (2003), Simon Williams (2005), and a handful of other anthropologists and sociologists have begun to construct a new integrative approach that conceives of sleep not so much as a time of asocial inaction, but as Robert Meadows (2005: 242) suggests, as a time of social interaction. No longer tied to the natural rhythms of light and dark, sleep today is constrained by the routines of work and social interaction and entails a complex series of negotiation with hosts of others regarding the regulation of sleep, and the conditions, locations, length, and social obligations under which it may take place. Ileen Montijn's (2006, this volume) explorations of the resistance of the Dutch working class to the adoption of new 'sanitary' bedding, Steger's (2003) work on negotiating sleep in contemporary Japan, and Smita Jassal's (2007) sophisticated analysis of the family and cultural dynamics of sleep in contemporary rural India, to name only three studies, explore avenues by which the study of sleep can be used to expose the sinews of social ordination, the expectations and desires involved in the micropolitics of daily life, and the cultural variability of a biological universal.

The possibility of a sociology of sleep, of course, necessarily implies the possibility of a history of sleep. The early eighteenth century was a period of remarkable social transformation in New England – a time when the impact of market forces, high rates of in- and ex-migration, and the first spasms of religious pluralism and sectarian competition began to resound, and in which the scars of the exuberant (and often bloody) sectarianism of the English Civil War were still fresh. Puritans, and many historians who have followed, often wrote about this period as a time of declension from the golden age of the seventeenth century, a period that witnessed a steep erosion of the intense communal and spiritual commitments that had bound the tightly knit, hierarchical theocracies of the founding generations.

More recently, however, the declension model has itself declined. Christine Heyrman (1984), among others, has argued that instead the social stresses besetting the region fuelled a sense of impersonal, external threat that may actually have reinforced the internal cohesion within maritime communities in Massachusetts. Rather than declension, New England villages seem to have experienced an intensification of the communal ideal and a creative social reformation. By examining aspects of religious discourse in the eighteenth century, I hope to sketch the 'overall logic' of early modern sleep, to use Peter Rensen's (2003) term, and to reveal the social and cultural context within which sleep was drawn into the protracted series of cultural negotiations such as adapted by New England societies, articulating basic conceptions of social order and obligation.

Nature's Soft Nurse

In speculation on the function of sleep at the turn of the eighteenth century, one can read the palimpsests of medieval and ancient hands. Sleep theorists continued to draw eclectically upon authors ranging from the omnipresent Aristotle to the medieval writers discussed by Gabrielle Klug (this volume), even as they integrated these ideas into a new anatomical and physiological framework for interpreting the nervous system. From Aristotle, early modern theorists borrowed a conception of sleep as a state characterised by impaired perception; a state best understood as enmeshed in a series of binaries that provided a peculiar structure for understanding its social implications – wakefulness was pitted against inattentiveness, activity against passivity, vigilance against vulnerability. Particularly later in the century, theorists argued too that sleep was highly variable in expression. The natural sleep enjoyed nightly differed only in degree, not kind, from sleep-like conditions such as trance, coma, ecstasy, reverie, and the mesmeric state, all of which were attended by more or less distinct phenomena ranging from dreaming to sleepwalking, sleeptalking, or sleep preaching.

But the tenor of sleep in the eighteenth century was set by its central role in the bodily economy, particularly in the maintenance of energy and vitality. As a 'perfectly periodical' function, in the words of the late-century naturalist Johann Friedrich Blumenbach (1795: 223), sleep occurred when 'all intercourse and communication between the mind and body' were suspended. As a person falls asleep, Blumenbach argued, a 'sluggishness and gradually increasing dullness of the external senses' overtook the body, 'together with a relaxation of most of the voluntary muscles,' followed in turn by a 'congestion of the venous blood in, and near, the heart' that led to the suspension of all '*animal* functions.' As sleep became 'complete,' only the vital bodily functions of pulse, perspiration, digestion, and the production of bodily heat continued, and these in a 'more sluggish and torpid manner' (Blumenbach 1795: 224). As the century neared a close, this physiologically based bodily economic interpretation of sleep increasingly rose to precedence.

Yet even at this late date, the term 'bodily economy' carried connotations that sat less than easily within a strictly physiological framework. In England and America, body and mind were widely considered to be bound inextricably by a pervasive and powerful force known as sympathy that drew like together with like (cf. Cox 2003). A dynamic and flexible concept, sympathy took on subtly different meanings in different ideological and intellectual milieus, and it could be regarded – sometimes simultaneously – as equally a physiological, social, or occult force (as much as these three registers were separate). Indeed, part of the power of sympathy lay in its ability to mean different things to different interpreters. For physiologists, sympathy could be invoked to explain how the immaterial mind controlled movements of the physical body and how medicine cured, and it could explain too how bodily parts without any discernable anatomical connection, for example, could display a common reaction to an external stimulus. For social theorists like Francis Hutcheson, David Hume, and Adam Smith, sympathy explained how a collection of individuals with disparate interests and origins could form a stable society, while for occultists, sympathy explained how the moon and stars – or angels and demons – shaped human behaviour or how one person could read another's mind. To say merely that these three registers were not mutually exclusive would be to miss the creative blend of alternative rationalities and epistemological approaches that characterised Enlightenment thought.

The world in which sympathy operated was shot through with hidden (perhaps occult) connections, and at least for some writers, it was a self-regulating, self-compensating world of correspondences in which mind influenced body, in which one body influenced another, and so on, anastomosing outward until one could imagine connections between a spiritual reality and natural reality, in which actions in the spiritual world were mirrored in the natural and vice versa. Sympathy was a powerful heuristic device, 'an immaterial principle of affinity or movement,' as the historian Ruth Leys writes, 'by which even the most distant parts of the universe might be drawn together' (Leys 1980: 7).

From this perspective, body and mind were often seen as a microcosm of the external world: a sympathetically bound, self-regulating economy of its own, with sleep providing 'refreshment and ease to both'. Body and mind were so 'wonderfully united', as the American physician Henry Rose (1794: 9) wrote, that 'the one may be affected by the other in reciprocal sympathy,' echoing Thomas Tryon's words of a century before, who theorised that it was the 'partial temporary Cessation of animal A[c]tions, and the functions of the

© Frank & Timme   Verlag für wissenschaftliche Literatur

external Senses' in sleep that enabled the individual to 'regain the strength of his body, and the faculties of his mind' (Tryon 1689: 12). Searching for an analogy to explain the process of energy recruitment, the popular writer John Trusler (1796: 96–97) suggested that the powers of mind could be likened to a current of water: 'if we want to give this water greater power,' he suggested, 'we dam it up, and when the water is run from the dam, if we wish to produce a fresh power, equal to the first, we shut the sluices, and collect the water again.' Sleep was akin to that shutting of mental sluices: the closure of the mind severing connection with the senses, and thus the external world, and permitting the body to follow suit.

But at the heart of this economy was a conundrum. The temporary severance of body from mind and the loss of rational control presented a challenge for theorists of any stripe. Particularly in the years after John Locke had instilled the senses into the foundations of natural knowledge, clergymen and physiologists were left to explore precisely what this severance implied about the 'balm of hurt minds' and 'chief nourisher in life's feast' (*Macbeth* 2.2.50–51), about what it meant to lose one's sensory connection to the natural world. Given that sympathy bound not only body and mind, but bodies and society, and societies in God, what could it mean to sever one's connection to the world around? To the divine?

Perilous Sleep

In New England, as elsewhere in the eighteenth century's English world, the response to these questions was framed within the context of large-scale transformations in American religious and civic life, with sleep providing an ideological resource for the ministerial elite in the project of (re-)forming an ideal, organically structured, naturally hierarchical society. Their writing on the purpose and nature of sleep is at once an attempt to come to grips with new social realities (sectarian competition, increasing secularisation, the advance of market forces) and an attempt to provide a map of a sympathetic social order.

Readily acknowledging the necessity of slumber, and even the pleasure, English and American writers weighed its corporal and mental benefits against social and spiritual obligations, discovering in sleep a daunting range of perils. The moral philosopher Henry Grove warned that unless carefully regulated, rest and sleep were 'not so properly *pleasures as indulgences.*' When engaged to its proper ends – 'to invigorate the body, [and] rally its scattered spirits' – sleep was a balm, but overindulged, it became a distraction from duty and work. God had implanted pleasures in natural lives to illustrate His bounty and glory, Grove insisted, but Grove warned against allowing pleasure to 'steal away *too great* a portion of our *time*, for we were not born for pleasure in this life, but for *labour* and *usefulness*' (Grove 1749: 317, 325).

That the utility of sleep was not simply a utility to the individual, but to the community, was abundantly clear. In his widely read *Whole Duty of Man*, the Royalist churchman Richard Allestree, adopted a functionalist approach like Grove, insisting that the benefits of sleep must be assessed relative to its aims. Rest and recuperation were divinely intended as preparation for renewed labour, 'to make us more profitable, not more idle,' and in the self-regulating economy of body and mind, too much sleep could easily result in damage to health or to mental well-being. After all, Allestree wrote, humans provide 'rest to our Beasts,' not because their idleness is pleasing, 'but that they may do us the better service.' Similarly, in his early critique of slavery, Thomas Tryon stressed the value of proper sleep and rest for slaves as a means of increasing profitability to the master. Given a midday rest, he argued, a slave 'shall thereby be rendered so lively, lightsome and brisk, that he shall be able to perform more labour than another man of the same natural strength, that is kept to it all day long' (Tryon 1684: 95–96).

Sleep, in other words, fulfils a vital economic function to match its physiological and (collective) spiritual functions: the bodily economy emerges as microcosm of the social economy, the recruitment of energy feeds a recruitment of economic vitality. In sleep, Allestree insisted, a person 'wastes his time' (that 'precious talent which was committed to him by God to improve'), 'injures his Body,' and injures his soul – 'not only in robbing it of the service of the Body, but in dulling its proper faculties, making them useless and unfit for those employments to which God hath designed them' (Allestree 1706: 203–204). The properly regulated bodily economy, in other words, becomes essential to the proper functioning of the formal economy, with self-discipline mirroring the discipline imposed by social superiors (slave masters, parsons). Undisciplined, immoderate sleep – the 'sure bane of thy outward Estate' – ensured that 'the sluggish person shall never thrive.' Indeed, to all appearances, it would be hard to conclude that the 'sluggard,' a person separated from the economy and society of this world, was alive at all. 'Sleep you know is a kind of

   © Frank & Timme   Verlag für wissenschaftliche Literatur

Death,' Allestree wrote, 'and he that gives himself up to it, what doth he but die before his time?' (Allestree 1706: 211).

This death, this separation from economy and society, was the prime concern for many of the Congregational clergy of New England. Almost by definition, the insensibility and loss of rational control inherent in sleep confounded that most Protestant command: the personal, rational commitment to apprehending scripture. For the clergy exploring the implications of sleep, metaphor frequently bled together with the social act, the two viewed as corresponding facets of a conjoint reality. After Bostonians were shaken from their beds by a powerful earthquake in 1728, for example, Samuel Wigglesworth saw the physical sleep of his parishioners as reflective of a deeper spiritual condition. The 'moral Sleep and carnal Security' into which too many had fallen, he claimed, had deadened their senses to the danger that should have been evident all around. 'Were we not putting the evil Day far from us?,' he asked (rhetorically, of course), 'hardening our Hearts, searing our Consciences, and walking in the ways of our Hearts, in Rioting and Drunkenness …, and all kinds of sensual Indulgences; without a Thought that for all these things God would bring us into Judgment?' (Wigglesworth 1728: 29). For Wigglesworth and his peers, sleep represented a condition of cosmic unguardedness. Left undisciplined, it represented a distraction from the engagement of mind and heart in the soul's duty at best, and more likely a subversion of spiritual preparation and a dereliction of one's spiritual duty to the community.

Cotton Mather drove this nail deeper, warning his parishioners to guard against sloth and sluggishness of mind by implying that sleep was not simply a passive unguardedness, but an active threat. It was 'ANOTHER of the *Thieves*,' Mather wrote, 'which makes People Snore away the *Time*, that should go to *Work* which GOD calls them to'. He exhorted his flock to shake off the 'Fetters of Immoderate Sleep, Oh! Seasonably shake them off,' and take up the vigilance that was sleep's antithesis. Even those who regarded themselves as awake, he warned, could not truly be sure of their spiritual safety, for 'Some awake,' he wrote, 'yet do fall asleep again' (Mather 1721: 13). Azariah Mather, a relative of Cotton's from Connecticut, concurred, warning that one often finds persons who seem to awaken when prodded, 'but no sooner is your back turned upon them,' he insisted, 'but they lie down to Sleep again.' So it is with slumber and the soul. 'Ah! How many are met with at a Sermon and are startled and alarmed,' Mather wrote, 'but before the next Opportunity are as fast asleep as ever? […] Some live almost all their days under Awakenings, but yet never awake thoroughly and to Saving purpose. They may awake, yet *not from the dead*, stand up and live' (Mather 1720: 4). Just as one could never be certain of one's election, one could never relax one's vigilance.

For an eighteenth-century audience, the impact of jeremiads on the uncertainties and covert dangers of sleep would have been intensified by the common experience of physical vulnerability at night, the feeling of spiritual vulnerability serving as counterpart to the bodily vulnerability experienced in the hours of darkness (cf. Ekirch 2005). In both cases, the senses – the means by which true knowledge was obtained – were impaired, but with senses closed and the rational mind subdued, the sleeping body was, if anything, even more prone to external attack than the physical. The inimitable Cotton Mather terrorised his fellow Bostonians with depictions of the perils that awaited them when sleep fell, and like darkness, palsied their spiritual senses. Every night, he insisted, defamers and devils and the 'Black birds of Hell' stalked the world, seeking to 'prevent the word the *Seed* of the *Word*, from getting well into the *Hearts* of the poisoned People.' These diabolical agents 'do it,' he argued,

> *by making us* Drowsy *and* Sleepy, *when the* Word *of God should have the Respects of a wakeful Attention paid unto it [...] From a Man that is* Asleep, *any thing may be taken away. When the Devils have lulled us* Asleep, *they may, and they do, take away from our Hearts, the good* Seed *of the* Word.' *Spiritual learning and spiritual profit is always contingent, always threatened. 'Oh! That we were more on our Guard!,' he exclaimed, 'Awake, my Friends, Awake; And let us Charitably jog, and pull, and* waken *one another! The* Philistines *of Hell are upon you! A Satanic Opium is administered unto you, by those Fiends of Darkness; who have a Plot on you, to deprive you of a* Word, *that might* Save your Souls'. *(Mather 1727: 35–36)*

It would be difficult to overemphasise this threat.

> *A Sinful Sleep, is indeed, a* Deadly *Sleep;'* Mather contended, '*it is a stupefying, and a venomous Bed of* Night-Shade, *whereupon men ly when they Sleep in Sin [...] If a man* Sleep, *he makes himself a prey to all his Internal and Infernal Adversaries; he lays himself open to all manner of Blows upon his Interests.*

© Frank & Timme   Verlag für wissenschaftliche Literatur

To Mather, the devil might well be the ultimate Protestant, the perfect counterpart to the vigilant Christian: never sleeping, never deprived of his rational mind, unflinchingly devoted to his business, unceasingly energetic in its pursuit. As we sleep, Mather warned, the devil was ever diligent, ever ready 'to throw his Nets over You; and You are *Hagridden*, by the most ugly things Imaginable,' he wrote. 'You are Sleeping; but I tell you [...] While you are *Sleeping*, your *Damnation* is *Hastening*; You are to Day, nearer to Hell, by Twenty four Hours than you were Yesterday.' Putting a fine point on his rhetorical bludgeon, Mather concluded: 'We are none of us very far from a *Night*, when we shall *Sleep in the dust*; We Shall not *Sleep in our Sin*, if we are duly Sensible, how sure, and how near, this *Night* is unto us' (Mather 1692: 17, 54, 56).

Foremost among the net-casting devils Mather had in mind were surely the 'enthusiasts,' the false religionists and extreme sectarians who had been the bogeymen of religious minds since the strife of the English Civil War. An all-purpose invective, the label enthusiast could be applied to any believer who stood outside the orthodox community and claimed religious inspiration of their own, and could be hauled out in disputes within congregations over the right of interpretation, and especially in disputes between orthodox Old Light Congregationals and New Light Evangelicals, and with either in disputing with any variety of other sects. For religious disputants on any side, sleep and its phenomena became a powerful tool in circumambulating the boundaries of appropriate religious discourse and excluding the enthusiasts, zealots, and delusives outside the pale of community.

Writing nearly a century after Mather, Benjamin Bell, a Congregational minister from Connecticut, argued that sleep was a time of deception, and given the tendency to wish-fulfilment in dreams, it was a time in which personal desire and the undisciplined senses ran amok. Just as sleepers faced the constant threat of 'wicked persons' at night, the spiritual sleeper was prone to enthusiasts and 'false teachers' who intended to cheat them of 'truth' and rob them 'of their most precious treasure, viz. an inheritance among the saints in light.' In sleep – natural or spiritual – illusion, delusion, and deception ramified. Natural sleepers have eyes, Bell remarked, 'but they see not [...] Altho' they are surrounded by the most beautiful objects in nature, yet can they discern none of their beauties.' Sleepers think, 'but their thoughts are frequently very irregular, and confused, and not agreeable to the truth;' they are capable of hearing, but the sound has no effect upon them; and they may talk in their sleep, 'but then what they say is frequently very foolish, and incoherent.' Sleep disrupts, and perhaps inverts the normal waking order. Sleep talkers 'rarely know what they say;' he wrote, 'they sometimes say one thing, and mean directly the reverse; their thoughts and words do not correspond' (Bell 1793: 8–9, 3–5). At the most fundamental linguistic and perceptual level, all sleepers were enthusiasts and sleep could be counted as a threat to the rational order, to the spiritual and civic as well, a threat to the economy, a threat to communication between the divine and mortal creation.

To address these threats, a well-regulated, vigilant society was demanded, guided (no doubt) by an erudite and active clergy whose task it was to interpret the Word properly. The vision of society that emerges through their sermons is an anachronistic one, to be sure, and surely more prescriptive than descriptive, recalling a unified Puritan New England bound in an intense communal solidarity. Spiritual and communal security were intertwined, both demanding active engagement and personal commitment to the communal project of salvation. Increasingly Mather suggested that god had commanded the proper Christian, each individually, to be like a watchman, always alert for mortal (and moral) peril. 'For a Watch-man to be found Sleeping is a sad thing,' he wrote. 'All Christians are appointed Watch-men, therefore should be careful that the Lord may not find them Sleeping at His Coming' (Mather 1709: 60).

Echoing Mather, Bell insisted that there was a need not merely for self-discipline in avoiding spiritual (and physical) sleep, but for social monitoring, a need to rouse those in the community who had fallen (asleep) as well as to rouse ourselves. It was the duty of ministers to guide, and of the community to awaken their fellows, Bell wrote, and it was the duty of 'sleepy dead sinners' to awaken when they 'see others awaking, and marching onward to the heavenly Canaan.' Sleepers 'ought to awake,' he insisted, for 'so long as they are asleep and dead, they are no benefit, *actively and designedly*, to GOD'S moral system.' The spiritual engagement demanded by god was to be spread throughout the civic order. 'We do not pretend to say that wicked men never make good members of society, good civil rules, and good politicians,' Bell surmised. 'We dare not say (as some affirm that other ministers have said, viz.) 'that no man ought to be invested with a civil office, but true Christians.' Tho' it must be acknowledged that a gracious and honest heart is one of the best qualifications in a civil ruler, yet GOD hath made even heathen kings, and such as were void of the true knowledge of GOD, instruments of great good to his church and people' (Bell 1793: 18, 16–17).

Sleep and Death

To understand the urgency in clerical assaults on sleep and their demands for vigilance and engagement, it will be helpful to take a closer look at the claims in several sermons that sleep is a species of death. This analogy (or identity), according to Cotton Mather, was 'easy, natural and very extensive.' At the simplest level, sleep functioned as a *memento mori*. The annihilation of sensation in sleep was so similar to the annihilation of death that every night, one invariably confronted the fact, as Mather insisted, 'that the *Night* of *Death* is hastening.' Such considerations ought actually to relieve Christians of the fear of death, he claimed. One would never grieve if an ailing friend entered into sweet sleep, nor would the true Christian grieve at death. 'What an Anodyne is this to Compose a Sorrowful Mind,' Mather wrote. 'We may say, *He is not Dead, but Sleepeth.*' For him, 'Death to the Faithful, is a SLEEP,' the latter preparing the natural sleeper for additional toil, the former preparing the spiritual sleeper for resurrection and the day of judgment, but both ending in a sweet and refreshed awakening, ending in a new life and new preparation for the duties and labours of an active Christian (Mather 1712: 1, 5).

But this optimism, if death can be called optimistic, was tied to another specific parallel between sleep and death: the putative liberation of the soul in both states from bodily constraint. Samuel Whitman, a Harvard-trained minister from Farmington, Connecticut, was adamant that scientific reasoning corroborated the notion that 'the soul,' as he put it, 'is capable of existing, *and performing its Operations, in a state of Separation from the Body.*' The soul neither slept nor swooned at death, as many implied, and never sat idle awaiting resurrection. 'It does not lie in a stupid and benum'd Condition like a Snake in winter,' he wrote, 'and wholly uncapable of performing its own proper Functions and Operations: a mere Fancy! a vain Dream!' Although many of his ministerial peers would disagree, Whitman's reasoning was clear. If the soul was reduced at death, insensate, he asked, would it not be better to remain in the infirm body, where one might at least have the comforts of god? It was logical to conclude that at death, the soul *'can live & act apart from the Body.* It has Faculties of its own, which it can Exert in its separate State' (Whitman 1727: 10).

Even in life, Whitman argued, experience showed that the soul can act independently of the body, 'as it sometimes does in Sleep when the outward Senses are lock'd up, and in Extasies and Trances.' The Patriarch Jacob was not so encumbered by his body that he could not commune with god and angels, nor was the Apostle Paul constrained during his heavenly raptures. While in the body, Whitman inferred, the human soul may exist in a state of separation from god, but when separated, he reasoned, it must then be 'present with the LORD, and enjoys communion with him' (Whitman 1727: 11).

Pursuing a similar tack, William Jones, the Rector of Pluckley, further parsed the relationship between sleep and death. Those who sleep might appear identical to the dead, he wrote,

> ... but then, in the case of natural rest, it is not the whole man, it is only the earthly part that falleth asleep: the mind is generally then most active and awake. It has a faculty of transporting itself to the most remote places in a moment; can be present with those whose absence it lamented in the daytime; and being as it were taken out of the body into the world of spirits, it can converse in imagination with those who have long since departed from this world, without being sensible that they are numbered among the dead. It is observed by most men, that in the time of Sleep they can think with more freedom, reason with more clearness, compose with greater readiness, and deliver themselves, upon any subject they are acquainted with, without that embarrassment to which the mind is subject, when it is weighed towards the earth by its attendance upon the functions of the body. (Jones 1772: 10–11)

Reliance upon natural senses alone was inherently limiting, Jones conjectured, and perhaps a sign of spiritual, if not cultural, inferiority. 'The knowledge of the heathen,' he argued, 'extended only so far as his senses would carry him; and therefore he sorrowed without hope, and *through fear of death was all his life-time subject to bondage*' (Jones 1772: 18). Based on his analysis, Jones concluded that the 'whole man' must never die, although the body may, and he added that once freed by death, the liberated soul experiences a greater freedom and activity than it ever did in the flesh. When the 'rational or animal soul' ceased acting over the senses, another physician argued, the senses were 'left at full liberty to act out their several natures, without being harassed by the various volitions of the mind' (Anonymous 1784: 8). Where this would lead was a new visionary terrain.

Visionary World

> *Now 'tis no wonder if a Discourse of such* sublime Subjects, *as the Enter-tainments of our Souls (during the Body's Nocturnal Repose) when they having shaken off for a time the Fetters of the Senses, are* upon the wing, *in the Suburbs of Eternity; of the* secret Intercourses of Spirits *with Humanity, and the* wonderful Communications *of the* divine *Goodness to his Servants in Dreams and Visions. (Tryon 1689: 3)*

Unfettered of the senses, and very much alive, the transport of the sleeper's soul laid open the possibility of direct divine revelation, one of the most sensitive subjects in eighteenth-century America. In England and America, as the historian Ann Kirschner (2003) has shown, a robust popular literature celebrated the visionary experience in sleep, the glimpses of heaven and hell and of this world and others it entailed. Yet while New Englanders had long yearned to set a match to the millennial fuse, the blasts of visionary zeal that periodically erupted from 'sleeping' visionaries were not always welcome. While even the most orthodox accepted that sleep represented a bodily state in which mortals could commune with the divine, fears of enthusiasm (false religion) had a dampening effect. Even those most disposed to accept the possibility of direct divine revelation – 'New Light' evangelicals, Quakers, Methodists, Free Will Baptists, Universalists, and Shakers among them – were keen to emphasise the sobriety, humility, and rationality of their dreamers, as well as their deference to authority (earthly and divine), thus insulating themselves against charges of toxic enthusiasm (cf. also Winiarski 2004; Juster 2003; Juster and O'Connor 2002).

The visions that descended upon sleepers in the eighteenth century spoke to topics as diverse as the Indian perspective on the Day of Judgment (cf. Anonymous 1773), the fate of the American Revolution (Clarke 1776), and the ultimate cause of the yellow fever epidemic of 1793 (Anonymous 1793), but the greatest number fell into a relatively narrow, even formulaic pattern: the spiritual journey to heaven and hell. The sight of lush green fields in the heavens, hosts of angelic beings clad in white, and divine music were *de rigeur*. While the visions might differ in doctrinal detail or eschatological speculation, visionaries from Anne Atherton in the 1660s onward reported over and over witnessing a serene spiritual landscape flooded by the sounds of 'Unparalleld Musick, Divine Anthems and Hallelu-jahs' and the sight souls of the departed ascending to be nearer God (Anonymous 1680: 2; see also Hill 1711, 1779; Anonymous 1710; Anonymous circa 1720).

Quite typically, sleeping journeys were highlighted by a cautionary trip to hell and a glimpse of glorious heaven itself, and quite often, of the Book of Life in which were inscribed the names of the elect (those who would ultimately reside in heaven). In 1741–1742, for example, an unidentified resident of Connecticut rode to heaven on the wings of a giant dove, flying past the yawning maw of hell before being taken by Christ himself and shown his or her name written in blood in the Book of Life (cf. Winiarski 2004). Similarly, the young New Yorker Sarah Alley witnessed a lake of lamentation and 'horrid pit' of suffering, as well as the 'place of happiness,' where sat Christ and his angels and many people 'clothed in white robes.' Alley's angelic guide entreated her, also typically, to alter her 'way of life and conduct, and to walk in the strait and narrow path' so that she might better prepare herself and (significantly) others to enter heaven. Christ himself commanded Alley to return to the world to 'warn the people thereof to repent and do better […]; and if the people did not repent and turn in the strait and narrow way, it would soon be too late, and they would fall in the lake that burns with fire and brimstone.' In sleep, at least, spiritual salvation remained a communal enterprise (Alley 1798: 7–9).

Most of the published dreams, according to Kirschner, were written by white men of lower social status, and among those whose denominational affiliations can be determined, most were evangelicals. Kirschner has argued that the majority of published dream narratives were 'noticeably restrained,' 'moderate' in tone rather than radical, and she argues in fact that they 'upheld authority more than overturned it' (2003: 216). One might argue, however, that quite apart from the content of the dreams, she underestimates the degree to which the experience of the visions themselves held a radical potential. Douglas Winiarski (2004) is more inclined to see a radical thread running through the spate of narratives from the period of the Great Awakening of the 1740s, but what seems likely is that idea that moderation is simply a rhetorical strategy on the part of the subaltern dreamers (and publishers) to evade allegations of enthusiasm – an effort to remain within the discursive community. As Winiarski has suggested, the very vision of the Book of Life struck at the Calvinist heart by providing infallible evidence of those who were assured of ascending to heaven, but it also contains a radical assertion of the right of spiritual self-interpretation. Claiming perfect and infallible knowledge of divine election was a challenge to clerical authority, of course, but here I wish to focus on less direct challenges, less direct transgressions of authority, emerging through the phenomena associated with sleep. Such resistance may not be as direct as the parishioners napping while Cotton Mather breathed fire, but they are claims that offer an alternative view of an ideal social order.

With reports of songs of praise 'which ravished my soul, and threw me into transports of joy,' the narrative of the Philadelphia Quaker, Thomas Say (Say 1792; Anonymous 1794; Watts 1774), bears a superficial resemblance to many heavenly voyages, yet Say centred his narrative far more on relations in this world and he was far more explicit than most in emphasising the continual connection, sympathetic and otherwise, between the departed and the mortal community. Leaving his sleeping body, Say reports, he witnessed the deaths of three local men in Philadelphia, two white (one of good repute, the other 'cast off') and one black, Cuffee, a slave of the widow Kearney. Peering from an alley into the widow's kitchen, Say saw all the details as Cuffee's body was laid out for burial, including an accident in which Cuffee's 'head fell out of their hands upon the board, about six inches, which I saw plainly.' Having left the impediments of the physical body behind, Say noted, he found that the walls of the house 'were no hindrance to my sight,' as transparent as glass. Long a supporter of education for black children and an antislavery advocate, Say commented that with his unfettered sight, he could see that as soon as Cuffee's soul appeared, 'it was clothed in a garment of unsullied white. I beheld him with joy' (Say 1792: 6–7). In death, at least, Cuffee was no longer chattel, no longer inferior. The specificity of the intercourse between living and dead, between natural and supernatural, that had been revealed through the medium of sleep was corroborated when the widow herself acknowledged that every detail of Say's account of Cuffee's death was on the mark, and his story was further corroborated when the deaths of the two white men he witnessed were confirmed.

Say's assertion that in sleep, the soul was liberated of the limitations of the body and senses was matched by assertions that the sleeping soul was freed of the constraints of space and time. Just as Say could see through solid walls, other visionaries reported remarkable phenomena in sleep, from mind reading to new modes of sensation. Freed of our 'present state of clouded existence' and of the limitations of social conditioning, this most solitary of nightly acts shed insight into the disproportion between the visible and invisible parts of creation, the material and immaterial, and it presaged the formation of an extended, highly integrated, truly sympathetic community (Anonymous

1798: 3). Remarkably, in the American context, as Say implied, this community could transgress the boundaries of race and social status.

Among all the effects of sleep, perhaps the most remarkable was its ability to illuminate the extensive, communal nature of perception itself, and few visionaries explored this interplay with more vigour than Heman Harris (Anonymous 1798). After conversing late one night with friends about the 'different modes of existence in the two invisible worlds', Harris wrote, he retired and 'fell into a deep sleep'. Believing he was near death, he felt 'stupid' for some time, 'till my increasing weakness, by degrees, locked up all my senses, and seemed to extinguish every faculty of my soul'. Leaving his corpse behind, much like Say, Harris discovered a range of new senses:

> *Before I was all dull, senseless, and dependent upon the organs of my body for every act of my mind; but now, independent of matter, I can range through the whole system without obstruction. Before, I received almost every conception from my eyes, my ears, and my other external sense, which were always languid and imperfect. But not my sight, my hearing, and all the perceptive faculties of body and mind, were reduced to this idea, that of thought. (Anonymous 1798: 6–7)*

As soon as he was 'independent of flesh and blood', Harris' perceptions began to intermingle 'with the very essence of whatsoever I formed an idea off'. As soon as he conceived of a thing, whatever it might be, he found himself 'by an inconceivable sympathy, instantaneously presented with it'. Whatever object came to mind, whatever place, was immediately made real, revealing, as Harris wrote, 'that length of time and distance of place, are things equally peculiar to the material world', but not to the world of sleep and spirit. Moreover, Harris was astonished to find himself 'surrounded, every where, by an innumerable company of thinking faculties', like himself, 'Immaterial, Immortal, Independent of Space'. Liberated of the body, shedding the tyranny of the mortal mind, he had entered into a new universe, an extensive community of sensation, a sympathetic community where all communicated by thought, rather than speech, and all experienced a 'continual interchange of [i]deas'. Although he seems not to have rejected the idea on principal, Harris denied only exchanging thoughts with god himself (Anonymous 1798: 7–8, 10).

Like many of his predecessors, Harris toured heaven and hell, and for all its idiosyncrasies and deviations from the orthodox line, he concurs with the

 © Frank & Timme   Verlag für wissenschaftliche Literatur

majority of his fellow visionaries in emphasising the theme of engagement and exchange. Heaven and hell, he wrote, were 'universally blended,' with 'good and evil spirits, promiscuously inhabiting every part of the universe,' differentiated immediately by their behaviours (like drawn sympathetically to like). The good were 'all love and benevolence,' the evil 'perfect hatred and malice.' The constant communion between the two, Harris suggested, served only to heighten the sense of punishment and despair among the wicked. Surprisingly, Harris found himself counted among the wicked. 'I was detested and shunned, with a heavenly detestation, by all the heirs of bliss,' he wrote, 'while I was treated, by those of my own order, with the utmost malice and insult.' So closed were his senses, however, that this condition had little impact upon him. 'I hated the Deity, with too much inveteracy, to be sorry I had counteracted his laws,' he wrote, 'and was too stubborn and inflexible to envy others the enjoyment of that happiness, which they were anxiously endeavouring to expect from the Almighty [...] I was too incorrigible, and too much transported with a desire of revenge' (Anonymous 1798: 7–9).

Such was Harris' hell, a separation from the society of the just and the benevolence of the divine, a wash of torment and pain. Such was sleep: a periodic separation form the world, a physiological necessary, a threat to body and soul, but an opportunity, if only fleeting, to engage in the deepest commerce with the structures of the universe, to commune with god and all humanity.

Conclusion

As both a biological universal and biological necessity, sleep was deeply ingrained in the culture of colonial New England, running as a leitmotif through a richly interwoven discourse on religion and morality, society and physiology. In many ways, the concerns expressed in that literature over the locus, form, and duration of sleep; when and how often it is indulged; and who may or may not partake bear some resemblance to the concerns identified in studies of cultures as far afield as ancient China, industrial-era Scotland, and contemporary Japan, the Netherlands, and India (Steger and Brunt 2003 eds). The constellation of social concerns embedded in classical Chinese literature, for instance, finds echoes among Anglo-American moralists, despite their radically different cultural contexts: concerns over the loss of control over one's rational faculties and the severance of social engagement echo from Beijing to

Boston, and so too concerns over the gentle hedonism of slumber, the loss of productivity (however measured), and the lack of self- and collective discipline (Richter 2003). Similarly, in colonial New England one can sense traces of the anxiety over the anonymity and social disorder of night that was experienced a century later in industrialising Glasgow, and one can sense too the intricate negotiations between authorities and those over whom they would bear their authority (Nottingham 2003).

Historians of the eighteenth century have often written of the efforts of orthodox (and to a certain degree, evangelical) religious writers to contain outbreaks of religious enthusiasm and constrain the content and interpretation of dreams and visions, but the contestation over religious dreams in colonial New England ran parallel to a separate and broader set of negotiations over the social, moral, and theological import of sleep itself. Quite apart from their efforts to quell the religious anarchy sparked by rampant dreamers (or sometimes to promote it), religious writers engaged with sleep's social and physiological dimensions, laying out a conception of sleep that imagined it as bearing both peril and potential. The comparison with early China here may be instructive. Antje Richter has shown that sleep in China was freighted with primarily negative connotations in Confucian and Legalist traditions whereas in Mohist writing it bore a 'positive counter-conception' (Richter 2003: 38).

In New England, however, the conception and counter-conceptions appear less easily separable by tradition, denomination, and social position. It was not so much that there are good and bad aspects to sleep as that the good and bad are inextricably intermingled, providing theologians and moralisers with a flexible and occasionally powerful instrument for delineating social and religious obligations, while simultaneously providing the mass of the sleeping public, as near as can be discerned, opportunities to stake their claim. Though always in need of regulation, proper sleep was a dynamic equilibrium between peril (of indulgence and absence of will) and potential (of spiritual and psychical insight). In that dynamic, social and religious expectations were hammered out on the anvil of biological need. In that dynamic, perhaps, one can sense the hand of unconsciousness crafting what conscious life entails.

Bibliography

ALLESTREE, RICHARD (1706) *The Whole Duty of Man, Laid Down in a Plain and Familiar Way for the Use of All.* London: W. Norton.

ALLEY, SARAH (1798) *An Account of a Trance of Vision of Sarah Alley, of Beekman Town, Dutchess County, State of New-York.* Poughkeepsie: Nicholas Power.

ANONYMOUS (ca.1680) *A Miraculous Proof of the Resurrection: Or, The Life to Come Demonstrated, Being a Strange But True Relation of What Hapned to Mrs Anne Atherton.* London: T. Dawks.

ANONYMOUS (1710) *The Sleepy Man Awak'd Our of His Five Days Dream.* London: Edmund Midwinter.

ANONYMOUS (ca.1720) *A Wonderful and Strange Relation of a Sailor.* London: s.n.

ANONYMOUS (1773) *A Strange and Wonderful Indian Dream, Dreamed on Cape-Cod, On the 14th of May, 1773.* Boston: E. Russell.

ANONYMOUS (1784) *Accurate and Complete Description of Sleep, In a Discourse Before the Medical Society, September 1782.* New York: for the author.

ANONYMOUS (1793) *A Dream, Dreamed by One in the Year 1757, Concerning Philadelphia.* Germantown: Peter Leibert.

ANONYMOUS (1796) *A Short Compilation of the Extraordinary Life of Thomas Say.* Philadelphia: Budd and Bartram.

ANONYMOUS (1798) *A Dream of Mr. Heman Harris, In His Last Sickness, a Little Before His Death.* Worcester: Leonard Worcester.

BELL, BENJAMIN (1793) *Sleepy Dead Sinners, Exhorted to Awake Out of Their Sleep and to Arise from the Dead.* Windsor: Alden Spooner.

BLUMENBACH, JO. FRED. (1795) *Elements of Physiology, trans. by Charles Caldwell.* Philadelphia: Thomas Dobson.

CLARKE, SAMUEL (1776) *The American Wonder: Or, the Strange and Remarkable Cape Ann Dream.* Salem: E. Russell.

COX, ROBERT S. (2003) *Body and Soul: A Sympathetic History of American Spiritualism.* Charlottesville: University of Virginia.

EKIRCH, A. ROGER (2005) *At Day's Close: Night in Times Past.* New York: Norton.

GROVE, HENRY (1749) *A System of Moral Philosophy*, vol. 2. London: J. Waugh.

HEYRMAN, CHRISTINE (1984) *Commerce and Culture: The Maritime Communities of Colonial Massachusetts, 1690–1750.* New York: Norton.

HILL, WILLIAM (1711) *The True and Wonderful History of Nicholas Hart: Or a Faithful Account of the Sleepy-Man's Visions.* London: Edward Midwinter.

HILL, WILLIAM (1779) *The Life of Nicholas Hart*, 3rd ed. Tewkesbury: s.n.

JONES, WILLIAM (1772) *A Disquisition Concerning the Metaphorical Usage and Application of Sleep in the Scriptures.* London: G. Robinson.

JUSTER, SUSAN (2003) *Doomsayers: Anglo-American Prophecy in the Age of Revolution.* Philadelphia: University of Pennsylvania Press.

JUSTER, SUSAN AND ELLEN HARTIGAN O'CONNOR (2002) 'The Angel Delusion of 1806–1811: Frustration and Fantasy in Northern New England', *Journal of the Early Republic* 22 (3): 375–404.

KIRSCHNER, ANN (2003) '"Tending to Edify, Astonish, and Instruct": Published Narratives of Spiritual Dreams and Visions in the Early Republic', *Early American Studies* 1 (1): 198–229.

LEYS, RUTH (1980) 'Background to the Reflex Controversy: William Alison and the Doctrine of Sympathy Before Hall', *Studies in History of Biology* 4: 1–66.

MATHER, AZARIAH (1720) *Wo to Sleepy Sinners*. New London: Timothy Green.

MATHER, COTTON (1692) *A Midnight Cry. An Essay For Our Awakening Out of That Sinful Sleep*. Boston: John Alden.

MATHER, COTTON (1712) *Awakening Thoughts on the Sleep of Death, A Short Essay on the Sleep, Which By Death, All Men Must Fall Into*. Boston: Timothy Green.

MATHER, COTTON (1719) *Vigilius, Or, The Awakener, Making a Brief Essay, to Rebuke First the Natural Sleep Which Too Often Proves a Dead Fly, in the Devotions of Them That Indulge It, and Then the Moral Sleep*. Boston: J. Franklin.

MATHER, COTTON (1721) *Honesta Parsimonia: Or, Time Spent as it Should Be ...* Boston: S. Kneeland.

MATHER, COTTON (1727) *Agricola, Or, The Religious Husbandman: the Main Intentions of Religion Served in the Business and Language of Husbandry*. Boston: T. Fleet.

MATHER, INCREASE (1707) *Meditations on Death*. Boston: Timothy Green.

MEADOWS, ROBERT (2005) 'The Negotiated Night: An Embodied Conceptual Framework for the Sociological Study of Sleep', *Sociological Review* 53 (2): 240–254.

MONTIJN, ILEEN (2006) *Tussen stro en veren: het bed in het Nederlandse interieur*. Wormer: Inmerc.

NOTTINGHAM, CHRIS (2003) '"What Time Do You Call This?" Change and Continuity in the Politics of the City Night', BRIGITTE STEGER AND LODEWIJK BRUNT (eds) *Night-Time and Sleep in Asia and the West: Exploring the Dark Side of Life*. London: RoutledgeCurzon, 191–214.

RENSEN, PETER (2003) 'Sleep Without a Home: the Embedment of Sleep in the Lives of the Rough-Sleeping Homeless in Amsterdam', BRIGITTE STEGER AND LODEWIJK BRUNT (eds) *Night-Time and Sleep in Asia and the West: Exploring the Dark Side of Life*. London: RoutledgeCurzon, 87–108.

RICHTER, ANTJE (2003) 'Sleeping Time in Early Chinese Literature', BRIGITTE STEGER AND LODEWIJK BRUNT (eds) *Night-Time and Sleep in Asia and the West: Exploring the Dark Side of Life*. London: RoutledgeCurzon, 24–44.

ROSE, HENRY (1794) *An Inaugural Dissertation on the Effects of the Passions Upon the Body*. Philadelphia: William W. Woodward.

SAY, THOMAS (1792) *A True and Wonderful Account of Mr. Thomas Say, of Philadelphia, While in a Trance, For Upwards of Seven Hours*. Philadelphia: s.n.

STEGER, BRIGITTE (2003) 'Negotiating Sleep Patterns in Japan', BRIGITTE STEGER AND LODEWIJK BRUNT (eds) *Night-Time and Sleep in Asia and the West: Exploring the Dark Side of Life*. London: RoutledgeCurzon, 65–87.

© Frank & Timme   Verlag für wissenschaftliche Literatur

STEGER, BRIGITTE AND LODEWIJK BRUNT (2003 eds) *Night-Time and Sleep in Asia and the West: Exploring the Dark Side of Life.* London: RoutledgeCurzon.

TAVES, ANN (1999) *Fits, Trances, and Visions: Experiencing Religion and Explaining Experience from Wesley to James.* Princeton: Princeton University Press.

TRUSLER, JOHN (1796) *An Easy Way to Prolong Life, By a Little Attention to What We Eat and Drink,* 4th ed.. Dover: Samuel Bragg.

TRYON, THOMAS (1684) *Friendly Advice to the Gentlemen-Planters of the East and West Indies.* London: Andrew Sowle.

TRYON, THOMAS (1689) *A Treatise of Dreams and Visions, Wherein the Causes, Natures, and Uses, of Nocturnal Representations, and the Communications Both of Good and Evil Angels, as Also Departed Souls, to Mankind, are Theosophically Unfolded.* s.n.

WATTS, ISAAC (1774) *The Visions of a Certain Thomas Say, of Philadelphia, Which He Saw in a Trance.* Philadelphia: William Mentz.

WHITMAN, SAMUEL (1727) *The Happiness of the Godly at Death.* New London: Timothy Green.

WIGGLESWORTH, SAMUEL (1728) *Religious Fear of God's Token, Explained and Urged.* Boston: D. Henchman & T. Hancock.

WILLIAMS, SIMON J. (2005) *Sleep and Society: Sociological Ventures into the (Un)known.* London: Routledge.

WINIARSKI, DOUGLAS L. (2004) 'Souls Filled with Ravishing Transport: Heavenly Visions and the Radical Awakening in New England', *William and Mary Quarterly* 61 (1): 3–46.

Beds Visible and Invisible:
Hygiene, Morals and Status in Dutch Bedrooms

ILEEN MONTIJN

In the Low Countries, as in many cultures, sleep and sleeping arrangements have always had moral implications, not unlike food, sex and their respective social contexts. The sheer physicality and the connection with pleasure of these activities meant that they needed to be regulated. As in many other parts of the world, early rising and moderation in sleep (as recommended, for example, in German mediaeval texts: see Gabriele Klug in the present volume) and sleeping on hard surfaces, for example, have been recommended. Some connection between sleeping and health had also been perceived long before the nineteenth century. A popular Dutch medical handbook of the 1630s (Van Beverwijck 1634) has a special chapter on sleep, in which all sorts of advice is given, mostly inspired by Aristotle's precepts and the writings of Galenus, to do with digestion and blood circulation.

One of doctor Van Beverwijck's prescripts in connection with health is ordering his readers to close the window before going to sleep; sleeping under the open sky is not recommended either (no clear reasons are given for this). This is surprising to us as later authors tend to insist on fresh air (for example, *De ervarene*; Anonymus 1753, and from then on practically every household manual). As regards the rest of what we would call hygienic prescripts, the cleanliness of the bed and its surroundings is only mentioned casually by Van Beverwijck and other authors of his time.

Cleanliness itself, as recommended in household manuals, obviously has – through concepts such as purification – a strong connection with morality. It was, from the eighteenth century onward, much elaborated on in household books with respect to the maintenance of the bed. Here, we must not think in the first place of soiled linen, but of bedbugs, fleas and lice and the like. Lowering of standards here meant immediate victory for the vermin, leading to much physical discomfort – and worse, the world could tell from the bites, especially on women's and children's pale skin. Flea bites were a sign of bad housekeeping, and thus of bad morals. The connection between keeping up standards of cleanliness and those of morality has, of course, stayed until the present day: the 'good' housewife is the one who keeps a spotless house.

However, in Christian cultures, morality in sleeping habits has a different implication as well: it means, or meant, that men and women (and older children of different sex) should not share a bed, unless they were married. In the 'permitted' combinations co-sleeping was widespread in the Netherlands; having a bed to oneself was, for the majority of the Dutch population, an unobtainable luxury well into the first decades of the twentieth century. Children slept in the same beds in surprising numbers, domestic staff were expected to share, and even in hospitals up until the nineteenth century, the sick were put into beds intended for two as a matter of course. For married couples in the Netherlands, co-sleeping in one bed was the norm – even among well-to-do citizens – as popular print books of the seventeenth and eighteenth century indicate (e.g. De Brune 1624).

With time, however, the number of rooms designed for a single purpose in the houses of the well-to-do increased. Co-sleeping declined (with the notable exception of married couples) and a certain striving for privacy was on the rise. As from the second half of the nineteenth century, the houses of the well-to-do generally had some rooms solely designed for sleeping (Fock 1987: 199).

I will argue in the following that privacy in sleep (such as the luxury of having bedrooms in a house and/or a bed of one's own) is a kind of missing link between morality and status. The connection lies in the fact that beds are not only objects used for sleeping, but also pieces of furniture, and the same duality holds for bedrooms, where they exist.

In the arrangement and furnishing of houses, social status is inevitably an important, and for many even an overriding consideration. But for the majority of the Dutch, considerations of status with respect to beds and sleeping habits was a latecomer compared to the importance of other aspects of interior decoration. Well into the twentieth century, sleeping arrangements were simply pushed out of sight in order to enhance the respectability of the more representational rooms. Furthermore, status considerations as regards sleeping arrangements have, from the middle of the nineteenth century onwards, become interestingly bound up with hygienic/moral arguments. I hope to make clear that modern thinking about sleep and beds (and even the market for beds) in the Netherlands were indeed deeply influenced by developments in the latter half of the nineteenth century.

Four-poster Beds, Box Beds and Plain Beds

From the late Middle Ages up until the early twentieth century, the Dutch population which slept in beds at all used one of three types of beds for that purpose. The first and most desirable bed was the bedstead, *ledikant* or four-poster bed, later often called *hemelbed*. It was free-standing, at least on three sides, and essentially curtained all around. The amount of textiles (wool or silk, before circa 1850) needed for that purpose gave it much of its status, as textile was, in pre-industrial society and even after that, an expensive commodity.

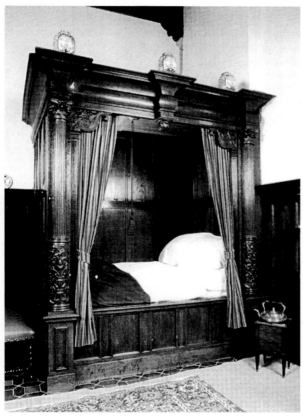

Fig. 1: Seventeenth-century box bed in Popta Castle, Marssum

The second type was not a bed at all, but a cupboard let into the wall or rather, into the panelling fixed to the wall – *nagelfest* as one says in German. The opening could be closed by a curtain or by doors. Box beds of this type, *bedstee* in Dutch, *Schrankbett* in German, *lit clos* in French, have existed in many societies throughout history. Given that the primary purpose of any dwelling was sheltered rest, it was often cheapest to integrate the bed into it while building, thus saving space and avoiding the need for a separate piece of furniture, and at the same time creating a relatively warm and draught-free space for sleeping. In the Netherlands, the box bed was widely used well into the twentieth century, especially in rural areas, but also in working-class housing. On the basis of interviews, literature such as novels, and a question-naire from 1983 sent out by the Meertens Institute for Social Anthropology, my estimate is that about half the population slept in them until around 1950.

The third, and in many respects the least-known type of bed was inherited from the Middle Ages: a plain, low, wooden bed, more than the others resem-bling our contemporary European beds: four legs, a frame between them, and on that, a sort of mattress; no curtains. It was used for staff in large houses, in attics and spare rooms, and variations of it were probably used by soldiers and prisoners, monks and nuns, but we know very little about it; surviving speci-mens from before the nineteenth century are difficult to date.

The free-standing, curtained bed and the box bed were generally about four feet (110–120 cm) wide, affording space for two persons at least; the modest, third type seems to have been narrower up until the nineteenth century. Only when it reached lower-class houses, it became wider in order to accommodate several people, resembling the box bed in size.

Bedrooms separate from living and reception rooms were not the custom in Dutch houses before the nineteenth century. As mentioned above, they were on the rise in well-to-do families. Traditionally, the free-standing, curtained beds used by the elite were often on display in the finest room even if, as the art historian C.W. Fock has demonstrated, in the eighteenth century some-times the owners of these beds used a different one (and sometimes even a box bed) for sleeping (C.W. Fock, interview 8 March 2005).

Engineers for Hygiene

The movement for housing reform in its first stages has been described as the 'hygienist movement'. The first major manifestation of this in the Netherlands was a report on the housing of the working classes in 1855 addressed to King William III by a special committee of the Royal Institute of Engineers. This institution had been founded in 1847 under the patronage of King William II. It concerned itself with modernisation in the widest sense, i.e. topics such as transport, sewerage, industry, and public health. The housing report was mainly concerned with sleeping conditions and health, and within that last aspect, fresh air. As is known, medical research had reached very definite conclusions about human need of oxygen, leading to strict quantitative rules about the amount of air – in cubic metres – required theoretically for each person in a house.

But these efforts, whether they made sense or not in modern medical eyes, were also – and fairly explicitly – connected with questions of morality. We clearly see what Tom Crook has called an obsession with the distribution of dormant bodies (Crook 2004: 8). The idea of many people of various sexes and ages sleeping together in confined spaces (where obviously, fresh air was scarce) was more and more abhorrent to members of the middle and upper classes. In city slums, which were beginning to form even in Dutch cities at this time, such cramped conditions were obviously present.

Along with their poor ventilation, box beds had the problem that they were difficult to keep clean as it was always dark inside, which in the eyes of reformers made them even more suspect. Moreover, housewives tended to store all kinds of stuff in them in the daytime, thus keeping out of sight the clutter of clothes and much more.

The solution offered by the engineers, and subsequent social reformers, lay in the propagation of the third type of bed described above, namely, the curtain-less, free-standing bed. Of this, a new model was invented and propagated just at this time, namely, the metal bedstead. This tubular metal bed, with its air of modernity and hygiene, was indeed to become more and more popular – not so much with the classes with which hygienist efforts were especially concerned, but with the middle classes, far into the twentieth century. Air could circulate around it, and bedbugs could not hide in cracks as they did in wooden beds.

Of course, the engineers also favoured separate bedrooms, of which even a nuclear family needed three in principle: one for the boys, one for girls and one for the parents. This was simply out of the question not only for slum dwellers, but even for most of the working population as they could not afford such houses. The engineers saw that and compromised, offering descriptions of model apartments with two bedrooms or even one, and indeed box beds (a minimum of three of these was more practicable) for sleeping.

Nevertheless, the focus of housing reform for years to come was to be the abolition of the box bed and the propagation of what inhabitants often called 'naked beds'. Occasionally, as early as the 1850s, model apartments for the working classes were built in Amsterdam without box beds, and thus requiring 'naked beds'. In fact, this last type had only disadvantages for the tenants. First, the 'naked beds' had to be bought or rented; second, they were unattractive obstacles in a room usually shared by a number of people, and thirdly, they offered less shelter from cold or draughts for those who slept in them. Of course, people can put up with enormous discomfort if they are convinced that they are doing the right thing, but it took a very long time to convince the Dutch in this case. In several instances, box beds were later built into houses like these because otherwise people simply would not rent them.

In the years that followed the first report by the Royal Institute of Engineers, the movement for housing reform grew. More reports appeared, and both private and cooperative housing societies were founded in the cities. In 1901 a Housing Law (*Woningwet*) was passed by parliament instructing all major municipalities to formulate and enforce building regulations – among other things with respect to social and hygienic conditions. Guidelines were published on which these regulations could be modelled; they left much room for compromises (for example, a maximum of three persons per bed was suggested!) and local variations were consequently great. The new law also empowered municipal authorities to shut down and evacuate dwellings deemed uninhabitable. In any city, signs reading *Onbewoonbaar Verklaarde Woning* (quarters declared uninhabitable) were a familiar sight well into the 1960s and 1970s.

In the twentieth century, the efforts of the movement for housing reform were taken up by a growing number of household manuals and women's (and other) magazines. The importance of healthy and sensible living conditions was widely felt among the enlightened bourgeoisie, and also among leaders of cooperative societies, working men's unions and the like.

© Frank & Timme   Verlag für wissenschaftliche Literatur

Bedrooms or Parlours?

The willingness of people to sacrifice comfort for their convictions was demonstrated in this period by another topic in social housing, for example, that of the parlour or salon, a 'nice room' used only for special occasions. Clearly, there was a very great desire for this in both working-class and peasant families as soon as their income rose above the barest minimum. Already at the building of the Netherlands' first housing estate, the so-called garden city of industrialist J.C. van Marken in Delft (1885), there were debates about this: the employees, and especially their wives, fervently desired such a parlour. (The other thing they desired was a small corridor which would prevent visitors from entering the house through the kitchen. In this last issue the tenants won, but not as regards to the parlour.) In the eyes of reformers, it was a familiar 'problem' that people would live all week huddled together in a smallish kitchen, so as not to touch and soil the parlour which was only entered on Sundays. They held, of course, that members of the lower classes did not need, and thus simply were not entitled to the luxury of such a reception room.

In working-class dwellings, the parlour and the bedroom were in direct competition for space. When in the 1850s in a famous Amsterdam working-class housing project, the Planciusblok, accommodations with a separate bedroom were built, many tenants preferred to turn this second room into a parlour, which was more important to them than a bedroom. The enlightened social reformers took their lessons from this undesirable tendency towards respectability and, in the next building project, installed toilets in the spare bedroom (remember, at this time these were not flushing toilets but simply barrels in a closet, and thus a very smelly and unpleasant addition to any room). This, they thought, would preclude their use as parlours. Apparently they did not object to families sleeping next to a toilet.

The desire for a parlour and the unwillingness of the working class to sacrifice their box beds both stem from the same desire, viz. to separate the private sphere from that of social representation, even in their own small dwellings. As long as one had box beds, the business of sleeping could be hidden away behind its doors, and a parlour was the first priority. The long-lasting popularity of the box bed, I think, can be explained this way.

The Appeal of the Alcove

The social reformers who wanted to get the Dutchmen out of their box beds found yet another obstacle in their way: the *gesunkene Kulturgut* of the alcove. This narrow, windowless room, or rather large *niche* in which to put a free-standing bed, had become popular in the upper classes all over Europe in the seventeenth and eighteenth centuries. It was actually a nice interior decorator's trick to create variation in a room, and give the owners of beds – which until then in the Dutch upper classes had been displayed in large rooms used for receiving visitors – a sense of intimacy, while at the same time the alcove as a whole could be displayed. And thus, perhaps, the rise of the alcove can be seen as a first step towards the specialised bedrooms, which only really emerged in the nineteenth century.

By the nineteenth century, alcoves were widespread among the middle classes. However, towards the end of that century they were on the way out, with one major exception. In lower-middle class and working-class housing in large cities, alcoves underwent a subtle transformation from about 1870 onward. In narrow apartments, which ran from front to back in deep buildings, an alcove was placed in the middle between the two rooms and became a tiny, windowless bedroom, usually with two box beds in it instead of free-standing beds.

Needless to say, alcoves, which (due to their aristocratic provenance and use of slightly more space) afforded more status than plain box beds, when used by lower middle classes were decried as unhygienic and pockets of foul air just the same. On the other hand, they became at least as popular as the traditional box bed. In the 1920s, a time of great housing shortage, when government subsidies were given for the building of working-class housing blocks, they were in frequent use. Hygienist objections against alcoves led to the exclusion of apartments with alcoves from subsidies, but there were debates on the question of whether apartments with alcoves could really not be subsidised, as they were so much in demand. A socialist alderman in Rotterdam in 1921 resigned over this issue, and it was not until 1937 that the city of Rotterdam explicitly banned alcoves in its building regulations (Prak 1991: 177–178).

Type I

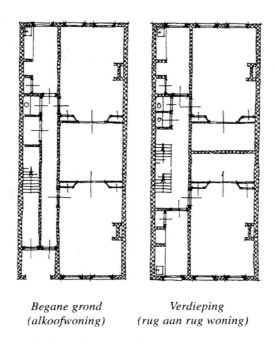

Begane grond   *Verdieping*
(alkoofwoning)   *(rug aan rug woning)*

19ᵉ-eeuwse woningbouw in grote steden

Fig. 2: Basic types of alcove flats, popular in Dutch cities c. 1850-1900. Left: ground floor flat with two rooms divided by an alcove. Right: two one-room flats with alcoves on upper floors.

In 1983 the Meertens Institute for Social Anthropology did a survey in which participants (mostly of rural background, but also some of urban provenance) of about 70–80 years of age were interviewed about beds and sleeping habits in their childhood, i.e. mainly during the years 1915–1930 (I evaluated this unpublished survey of about 120 only qualitatively, not quantitatively, as the material is quite patchy). A clear majority of respondents mentioned box beds – a minority of which were situated in alcoves. Usually two persons (parents or children) slept in a bed. Surprisingly, hardly any of the respondents mentioned lodgers or live-in grandparents. The only non-related household members mentioned were domestic staff. They slept in box beds, while their employers, well-to-do farmers in the province of Groningen, used twin beds, which I will elaborate on in the following.

But the movement away from the box bed had obviously begun in the early 1920s; several respondents to the Meertens Institute survey mention their parents stopped using box beds at this time, or their families sleeping in free-standing beds despite the presence of box beds. These cases come from educated families – the struggle can be seen in a headmaster's family in rural Groningen, where in principle everyone slept upstairs (meaning, in plain beds) and the three downstairs box beds were only used in case of illness, for over-night visitors, and for storage, respectively.

In 1960, the removal and/or conversion of box beds in old working-class apartments was still an issue in housing and interior-decoration advice, as is illustrated by an article in the seminal modernist magazine in this field, *Goed Wonen* (the title of this magazine is difficult to translate into English: *Good home decoration* might be somewhere near, but the undertone is one of 'proper living').

Folding Beds and Twin Beds

Two alternative forms of beds, both developed in the nineteenth century, had emerged by the twentieth century which both also occur in the Meertens Institute survey, viz. the folding bed and the *lits jumeaux* or twin beds. Both innovations were taken up by educated and/or well-to-do families.

Folding beds were invented as a solution to cramped housing conditions and propagated, for example, in industrial exhibitions in the nineteenth century. But as these folding beds in their early stages were rather complicated and thus expensive contraptions, they were not used by the lower classes for whom they were intended, and remained rare. The modern folding bed made of tubular steel, hidden in a wooden casing which made it look like a low, cur-tained bookcase in its upright position, appeared in the 1920s. In the Meertens Institute survey, we see folding beds used by a small family in Amsterdam, where one is placed in an alcove for a single child, and another one – typi-cally – in an architect's family in a private house in a rural town, where three children have folding beds in their own rooms. This use of folding beds in children's rooms in order to obtain more space for playing in the daytime was propagated by progressive architects and interior decorators from the 1920s (for instance, the striking, world-famous Rietveld-Schröder house in Utrecht, built by pioneer architect Gerrit Rietveld in 1925, sported them too).

Folding beds reached their greatest popularity around the middle of the twentieth century, in the 1950s and 1960s when there was a great housing shortage which was not, like earlier, connected with abject poverty. Now, people were able to spend some money to make the best use of limited space, while box beds were definitely on their way out, and were not being installed in new houses. Here, we actually see a continuation of something which I mentioned earlier, viz. the wish to create a room suitable for representative purposes – in other words: the display of social status – in family homes. Beds and the paraphernalia of sleeping needed to be banned from these 'nice rooms' – not for hygienic, but for social reasons. Anyway, folding beds were not particularly hygienic in themselves, as some advisors pointed out, because the bedding was stowed away in an airless cupboard in the daytime. But where there was a choice between hygiene and representation, the latter won.

Lits jumeaux or twin beds (i.e. adjoining single beds) for married couples were also a nineteenth-century innovation. It coincided with the development of the bourgeois bedroom into a separate, very private space used for sleeping, but also for grooming oneself, for washing, getting dressed, and other private activities such as letter writing. These rooms were often elaborately furnished, in blatant contrast with the recommendations for hygienic bareness given in manuals for the furnishing of bedrooms of the working classes. Twin beds, consisting of two single beds pushed together, in the early stages sometimes dressed up with curtains and an awning to resemble an old-fashioned bedstead or *ledikant*, are reputed to have originated in France, where King Louis-Philippe, the bourgeois king, seems to have taken them up with his wife Marie-Amélie. In royal circles, the co-sleeping of man and wife was an innovation. Among the Dutch bourgeoisie and probably elsewhere too, twin beds were a kind of status symbol. They took up more space and needed more sheets and blankets than an old-fashioned four-foot-wide bed for two.

But the fashion for twin beds was also fed by the hygienically tinted idea that it was somehow better and more respectable to sleep in adjoining single beds, than to huddle together bestially in one larger one (as did the lower classes, of course). While the elaborately furnished bourgeois bedroom at last fell out of favour in the 1920s, recommendations for twin beds – as opposed to double beds, plain beds wide enough for two – can be found in modern manuals on interior decoration up until the 1960s, and, for example, in the magazine *Goed Wonen*: 'The double bed cannot be regarded as a satisfactory place for sleeping' (*Goed Wonen* 1950 [March]: 134). In a major survey on Dutch households held by the large electricity company Philips in 1957 (*De Nederlandse huisvrouw* 1958), there turns out to be a clear connection between family income and sleeping in twin beds, although even in the wealthier group, this was used by just one quarter of the respondents.

In present-day beds, the distinction between double and twin beds is almost mute, as twin beds, in spite of having become 160 or even 180-cm wide, can be connected and even made up as one, so that the split between the two is almost imperceptible. Most Dutch couples nowadays use twin beds rather than double ones, and would probably argue that there are practical advantages (when moving the bed about for instance) and they also have the convenient option of being able to raise the heads of each bed independently without interfering with the other. But I wonder if the tradition does not stem from the status of the *lits jumeaux* several generations earlier.

Hygiene and Respectability

The movement for housing reform has had considerable influence on the shaping of working-class housing in the decades around 1900. On the other hand, I think that its *direct* influence in the disciplining of sleeping habits has been overestimated in recent anthropological and social-historical literature (e.g. Cieraad 2006). Of course, here and there, housing inspectors did invade the dwellings of the working classes in order to discipline sleeping arrangements. But this was only a minor, illustrative episode in the history of housing and social disciplining in this period.

The really significant invasion of the private sphere (including bedrooms) was more subtle, and it ultimately concerned almost the entire population. The development I am trying to outline in this chapter runs roughly as follows.

First (from circa 1850) hygienists tried to chase the lower classes from their box beds. This, however, could only be realised at the cost of privacy, and so the campaign was not very successful. Privacy was closely connected with social status, i.e. the need for representational spaces without beds. The lower classes, when confronted with the choice between hygiene and privacy/social status, chose the latter.

In contrast, in the upper classes, hygienic standards were easier to follow as, in larger houses, they were easily combined with the growing need for privacy. For the bulk of the population, this only became possible towards the middle of the twentieth century. Then, considerations of hygiene – and even a kind of 'medicalisation' of beds which at first appealed only to the bourgeoisie – could turn into a matter of respectability: of knowing how to make sensible choices in one's home.

The whole process fell in with the rise of the general civilising campaign which, taken broadly, lasted nearly a century starting around 1870. This campaign, in so far as it concerned material things like housing and home-making, was greatly helped by a substancial increase in wealth. Accompanying this, and all too easily overlooked, was the increase in the living space available for each inhabitant. All in all, this civilising campaign ultimately led to the bourgeoisification – *Verbürgerlichung* – of all but a small bottom stratum and an even smaller top stratum in Dutch society.

These are sweeping statements, the result of which for sleeping and bedrooms I should like to illustrate with a very palpable example. Namely, with the success of the Dutch company Auping (cf. Auping 1951) producing beds and especially, bed bases made of metal.

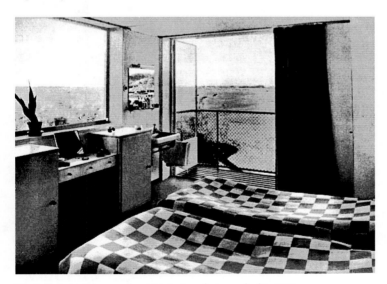

Fig. 3: Twin beds in a modernist interior, photographed in 1935.

Beds for Health

The Royal Auping Company was founded in 1889 by a blacksmith, Jan Auping, in the provincial town of Deventer. He invented a new type of bed base to be used in any kind of bed frame, consisting of metal coils twisted together in a mesh so as to obtain an exceptional springiness. This bed base was called a 'health mattress', although of course some form of mattress was still needed on top of it; this was usually filled with kapok up until the 1960s. But the flexible metal bed base (children could jump up and down on it as if on a trampoline) was the foundation of the Auping company which exists to this day, and has dominated the Dutch bed market for most of that time.

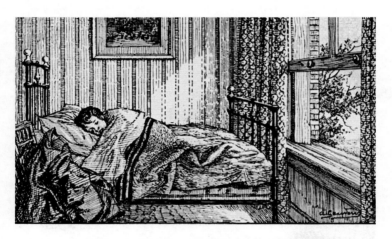

49. Slaap met open ramen!

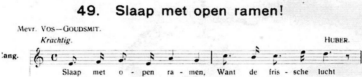

Fig. 4: Child in a 'hygienic' metal bed, sleeping with window 'hygienically' open; from a song book of 1921.

The first order of the company, in 1889, was for the beds in an Amsterdam hospital – one of a wave of new hospitals, as these previously rather squalid institutions were now turning into places fit not only for the poor, but for the bourgeoisie as well (though of course, not in one and the same hospital). The

© Frank & Timme   Verlag für wissenschaftliche Literatur

'health mattress' hygienic qualities, such as the fact that air could circulate freely through the mesh, were counted as a great advantage in Auping's product.

The combination of medical approval and remarkable comfort brought the company immediate success. Ten years later, Auping received an order for all the beds – dozens of them – for the Royal Palace in Amsterdam for the inauguration of the young Queen Wilhelmina in that city in 1898.

In its publicity, Auping has never ceased to accentuate the sound hygienic quality of its product, and hammered home the point that sleep was not a matter to be neglected. On the contrary, sleeping well was of the utmost importance for everyone, and required serious attention by experts, such as Auping and bed manufacturers.

One claim in their publicity between the world wars is of particular significance in that respect. It ran: *Auping keeps watch over one third, but the most important part of your life!* ('keeping watch' in Dutch is the same word as waking, i.e. staying awake, presumably to protect somebody who is sleeping, and therefore vulnerable). Dutchmen were told that the choice of bed was a serious matter, which was readily accepted. This was reflected in advisory articles and household manuals telling their readers not to choose just any pretty bed, but to act responsibly in this matter. And of course, such a 'sensible' choice could hardly be the cheapest one. Auping has always served what marketeers call the top end of the market, or at least the top half. There were a lot of cheaper imitations around, which they have always managed to keep at bay.

The success of Auping coincided with the great modernising campaign which swept though Dutch architecture and design in the interbellum up until the 1960s. The Dutch bourgeoisie was remarkably unanimous in its conviction that light, air and space were primary considerations in housing. Nowhere else in Europe, I believe (with the possible exception of some Scandinavian countries), was the modernist message so successful, and was the 'airless clutter' of the nineteenth century denounced with such fervour. One protagonist of this movement was the magazine quoted above, *Goed wonen*, with its view that sleeping in a single wide bed even for couples was to be rejected.

Because the upper classes had accepted hygienist precepts so much earlier and more thoroughly (due to the fact that they had the means), hygienist considerations – and even a kind of 'medicalisation' of beds which at first appealed only to the bourgeoisie – could turn into a matter of respectability for the whole population. This entailed the readiness to pay a relatively high price for a 'good' bed (which echoes the classic willingness of 'responsible', i.e., socially ambitious members of the working class to pay higher rent for their apartment, because they know of the importance of the surroundings where one raises one's children).

In the last fifteen to twenty years, housing, and interior decoration in particular, have become extremely important to a large segment of the Dutch population. Bedrooms have received an unprecedented amount of attention, and are subject to decoration as never before. Auping has been suffering serious competition from other bed manufacturers of foreign origins. Two Swedish companies, Ikea at the cheap end of the market and Hästens at the high end, have emerged. The success of the latter, where beds cost anything up to 45,000 euros, is especially remarkable.

An Auping staff member trained as an anthropologist agreed with my suspicion that the Dutch market for beds is an attractive one, specifically because the Dutch have 'learned' to spend a lot of money on beds because of their importance for their health, hammered into their minds by Auping. After years of predominance of the mesh bed base, the current preference of consumers has turned towards box spring beds, the most expensive of 'sleeping systems' – and Auping itself has deviated from its own tradition by producing these, too.

But the message with which it attempts to sell its beds has not changed very much. In a recent newspaper advertising campaign, which must have been extremely expensive, the company's claims to improving the lives of its customers have increased fantastically. The motto of the campaign is: *Auping nights, better days*. And the text under a large photograph of their newest model, the Auping Superbox, runs as follows:

> *Better ventilation, better support, better adjustment. Better sleep, better rested, better mood, better aura, better meeting, better deal, better salary, better position, better car, better house, feeling better, better Daddy, better husband, better marriage, better food, better health, better looks, better love life, better sleep, better ventilation, better support, better adjustment, getting up better, better rested.*

This can, of course, be seen as a very contemporary attempt to make a bed part of something now called *lifestyle*. But what shines through is a cocktail of age-old notions about health, morals and social status which originated somewhere in the latter half of the nineteenth century, and which has deeply affected Dutch thinking about sleep and beds.

   © Frank & Timme   Verlag für wissenschaftliche Literatur

Bibliography

ANONYMUS (1795) *De Ervarene en verstandige Hollandsche Huyshoudster* (The experienced and sensible Dutch housewife). Amsterdam: Gravius (second printing; first printing 1753).

AUPING, W.J.W. (1951) *Beknopte geschiedenis van Auping Deventer van 1868 tot 1951* (A short history of Auping Company at Deventer 1868–1951). Deventer: Auping.

BEVERWIJCK, JOHAN VAN (1649) *Schat der Gesontheyt* (The treasure of health) Dordrecht: Hendrik van Esch.

BRUNE, JOHANNES DE (1624) *Emblemata of Zinne-werck, voorgesteld in beelden, gedichten en breeder uitlegghingen* (Emblems or meaning, presented in images, poems and wider explications). Amsterdam: Jan Evertsen.

CIERAAD, IRENE (2006) 'Slaapkamergeheimen: een recente cultuurgeschiedenis van bed en slaapkamer in de Nederlandse woninginrichting' (Bedroom secrets: A short cultural history of beds and bedrooms in the Netherlands), *Medische Aantropologie* 18(1): 18–35.

COMMISSIE UIT HET KONINKLIJK INSTITUUT VAN INGENIEURS (1855) *Verslag aan den Koning over de vereischten en inrigting van arbeiderswoningen door eene Commissie uit het Koninklijk Instituut van Ingenieurs* (Report to the King on the demands and furnishing of working men's housing). Den Haag: Van Langenhuysen

CROOK, TOM (2004) 'Privatising Sleep: Bodies, Beds and Civility in Victorian Britain', ESRC-sponsored seminar series on Sleep and Society: Critical Themes, Future Agendas. Warwick: University of Warwick.

De Nederlandse huisvrouw (1958) (The Dutch housewife). Eindhoven: Philips.

FOCK, C.W. (1987) 'Wonen aan het Leidse Rapenburg door de eeuwen heen', P.M.M. KLEP ET AL. (eds) *Wonen in het verleden. 17e–20e eeuw* (Living in the past. 17th–20th century). Amsterdam: NEHA: 189–205.

Goed Wonen, Maandblad van de Stichting Goed Wonen (monthly magazine of the foundation for proper habitation) 1948–1969.

MONTIJN, ILEEN (2006) *Tussen stro en veren. Het bed in het Nederlandse interieur* (Between straw and feathers/springs. The bed in the Dutch interior). Wormer: Inmerc.

PRAK, NIELS L. (1991) *Het Nederlandse woonhuis van 1800 tot 1940* (The Dutch house from 1800 tot 1940). Delft: Delftse Universitaire Pers.

SCHADE, CAROL (1981) *Woningbouw voor arbeiders in het 19de-eeuwse Amsterdam* (Working man's housing in 19th-century Amsterdam). Amsterdam: Van Gennep.

A Bed for Two?
Gender Differences in the Reactions to Pair-sleep

G ERHARD K LOESCH AND J OHN P. D ITTAMI

Introduction

Cross-cultural anthropological studies have shown that group sleep with individual bedding is historically the most prevalent sleep environment in human societies (Worthman et al. 2002). Co-sleeping, on the other hand, defined as the sleep situation of two individuals with common bedding and close contact, is characteristic of mother-infant interactions in most societies. Although the duration of mother-infant co-sleeping is affected by culture and individual preference, it clusters around the first-week post partum, the consolidation of the infant's nocturnal sleep or the end of nursing. There are few examples of cultures with extended father-infant co-sleeping (Jenni and O'Connor 2005).

Co-sleeping with an adult partner is a more recent phenomenon restricted to certain cultures and even then often dependent on both the age of the individuals and their relationship. This sleeping arrangement, however, is characterised by some additional features: In contrast to the mother-infant sleeping arrangement, usually the whole sleeping phase of a pair is spent together. In addition, the sleepers are often emotionally engaged by the partner's presence and sleep may be accompanied by sexual activity. Therefore, the term 'pair-sleep' should be used for this particular sleeping arrangement. In some studies the term 'couple-sleep' has been used, to refer to the sleep of married couples or partners living in a long-term relationship. Couple-sleep is pair-sleep. However, we would emphasise that pair-sleep describes a more general phenomenon of both, homo- and heterosexual relationships, independent of the duration of the partnership. It is thus a better construct on which one can try to base generalities.

With the development of the media and its concomitant dominance in communicating social and cultural norms, pair-sleep as an expression of intact socio-sexual relationships in pairs has become a widespread phenomenon.

This change in sleep environment has also been paralleled by the consolidation of sleep into the night. Sleeping during the day has become more and more restricted. Today in many cultures, there is simply no time for naps, although in others napping is still popular (e.g. Steger 2004; Li Yi 2003; Brunt 2003). Driving forces in the expansion of the pair-sleep-in-couples phenomenon has also been the so-called 'triumph of monogamy' in human societies (Herlihy 1995). This is a social and economic phenomenon that has placed enormous importance on the socio-sexual bond between sexual partners and institutionalised marriage. It is also one of the most popular themes in entertainment. Sexual pairs are suppoosed to have intact, romantic relationships. Pair-sleep is a logical product of this development with possible compounding factors associated with paternal certainty and mate guarding. In some cultures the practice of pair-sleep is so pronounced that its expression is seen as an indication of the functional relationship between a husband and wife.

With these points in mind it is not surprising that the pair-sleep situation may not always be in the interest of the individual, even if it is a cultural norm. It is also common knowledge that bed partners are sometimes, or even often, disturbed by the sleep behaviour of their bed mate. Having a snoring partner is a common complaint and one reason for disrupted sleep in women (e.g. Hislop and Arber 2003). It is surprising that this situation has not been given more attention in sleep research. Sleep pathologies are widespread in Western cultures and sadly potential effects of the sleep environment on the development of sleep deficits have been overlooked. One explanation might be that couples usually do not complain about the sleep behaviour of their partner. Another explanation would be that researchers interpret this kind of sleep disruption as an isolated but perhaps recurrent phenomenon that is compensated for by recuperative sleep on subsequent nights. This would be similar to sleep restriction associated with work schedules where many sleep researchers bank on an individual's capacity to compensate for sleep debt on their days off (Wittmann et al. 2006).

The crux of the issue is that the pair-sleep situation and its accompanying negative effects on individual sleep patterns is probably as relevant in modern society as work-related sleep disturbances. The difference is that there may be less chance for recuperation for pair-sleep sufferers. For this reason it appeared imperative for us to determine first of all whether pair-sleep had an effect on sleep structure and second whether this effect was the same for both individuals in bed. Our greatest concern was that some individuals or pairs might feel unwell under these culturally dictated sleeping habits. Apart from this, there was the underlying fear that the reactions might be affected by the gender of the partner.

On the basis of the prevalence of pair-sleep and potential medical impact, we opted to study the phenomenon (see also Kloesch, Dittami and Zeitlhofer 2008). Empirically, it was difficult to collect data on sleep patterns in pairs that would shed any light on the issue. Forced separation or unification of bed partners produces artefacts that cannot be controlled for. Our solution was to address the issue by recruiting couples with stable relationships that regularly slept alone or with their partner. This is characteristic of some pre-marriage arrangements in Western cultures, but it is not common. The situation is similar to the ancestral sleep custom of group or individual sleep with occasional sexual contact and the additional component of spending the whole sleep phase together.

Stable pairs had the advantage that both partners were used to sharing one or the other bed so that we were able to examine the direct effects of bed choice on the reactions to partner presence during the sleep phase. The study required monitoring both individuals when sleeping alone and in pair-sleep situations. In addition, it was necessary to compare subjectively reported data of sleep diaries with objective data on actual sleep time, as recorded by wrist-worn activity monitors (so-called actigraphs). Finally, sexual contact in the sleep phase had to be treated as a confounding parameter in the analyses of sleep structure and quality. With these prerequisites is was possible to recruit ten heterosexual pairs for the study.

The Phenomenon and the Study in Question

The following report is based on an on-going study and a paper published by Dittami et al. 2007. The starting point was that both cultural and biological aspects to sleep can interact to affect human health and development (e.g. Jenni and O'Conner 2005). Although the biological need for sleep has not changed, the cultural dictates concerning sleep behaviour have undergone enormous local and temporal changes (e.g. Hicks and Pellegrini 1991; Iglowstein et al. 2003). The changes in behavioural norms have had an impact on both the subject's assessment of how and why we sleep and, the physiologically more relevant aspects of sleep environment and sleep times. Social dictates have then, in some cases, produced potential discrepancies between cultural sleep norms and the biological needs of individuals (Jenni and O'Connor 2005). Studies of these interactions have underlined the social aspects of sleep and their effects on sleep (e.g. Aubert and White 1959a and 1959b; Schwartz 1970; Gleichmann 1980; Taylor 1993; Williams 2005) and brought up the issue that cultural dictations of sleep customs may not always be in agreement with the individual's physiologically determined need for sleep.

In the past century two developments in adult sleep patterns should be of particular concern to sleep researchers and the medical community. One is the consolidation of sleep in nocturnal periods. Napping and afternoon rest phases have virtually disappeared in some societies. This has been proposed to be a consequence of the industrial revolution (Ekirch 2001) that changed the diurnal and nocturnal patterns of activity in large parts of the world. Another recent development is the habit of pairs to share beds to sleep in. This is actually a modern custom whose prevalence differs among cultures. It is assumed to have found its roots in European and their related North American cultures over the past century. Thus, in terms of cultural history, it is very recent. There are few data on its actual beginnings. Cross-cultural anthropological studies however have shown collective or group sleep with individual bedding and not pair-sleep as the most prevalent sleep environment in human societies (Worthman and Melby 2002). Pair-sleep with common bedding and close tactile and olfactory contact is primarily found in mother-infant interactions and not among siblings or in sexual pairs. As mentioned in the introduction, there are nonetheless very large differences in parent-offspring contact during sleep, ranging from no contact to maternal interactions and in some cultures even paternal contact (Wulff and Siegmund 2000; Jenni and O'Connor 2005). Due to the widespread acceptance of cultural norms propagated by the entertainment industry, the practice of pair-sleep has become very popular.

The potential effect of partner presence in a single bed over the whole sleep phase is an unresolved issue. Some researchers have recognised the potential problems in this context and proposed that pair-sleep involves so-called negotiations between the individuals whenever they sleep together (Meadows 2005; Meadows et al. 2005). Beyond the theoretical assessment, however, there have been few empirical studies to prove the assumption. About half a century ago there was a sleep laboratory study in which changes in polysomnographic sleep recordings with pair-sleep were documented (Monroe 1969). Although

© Frank & Timme   Verlag für wissenschaftliche Literatur

the effects were suggested to be greater in females, there were no direct analyses of sleep quality or efficiency associated with the study.

Since then, researchers have shied away from the problem because of difficulties in the experimental design and uncertainty about whether effects might have been caused by the partner. More recent developments in actigraphy (for an overview see Kloesch et al. 2001) enabled researchers to collect detailed information on sleep behaviour in the pair-sleep condition (e.g. Pankhurst and Horne 1994; Meadows 2005; Meadows et al. 2005). There were also studies on why couples sleep together. Other studies addressed the issue of movement and sleep synchronisation between partners in bed (Pankhurst and Horne 1994; Meadows et al. 2005), but less information was collected on the effects of the pair-sleep environment on the timing of sleep, sleep lengths, subjective sleep quality or possible gender-dependent reactions to partner presence (see review in Rosenblatt 2006).

As mentioned above, these effects were investigated in a study performed by our team in Vienna between November 2005 and July 2006. We enrolled young unmarried couples that had no children and no history of sleep disturbances. The subjects were ten pairs aged between 21 and 31 years; females were 25.7±3.56 years old and males 26.9±3.03 (mean value, standard deviation). No homosexual pairs applied for participation. The duration of the partnerships ranged from two to 78 months, with a median of five months. There were no consistent differences between the numbers of nights the female slept in the male's bed and those of the male slept in the female's. All subjects completed the Pittsburgh Sleep Quality Index (PSQI; Buysse et al. 1989), a standardised sleep history inventory and the Morningness-Eveningness Questionnaire (MEQ; Horne and Oestberg 1976) to evaluate morning or evening chronotypes.

The PSQI is a self-report scale that retrospectively measures subjective sleep quality of the previous four weeks. Twenty items are used for the quantitative measurement and are assigned to seven components (subjective sleep quality, sleep latency, sleep duration, sleep efficiency, sleep disorders, consumption of sleep aids and daytime fatigue). The total score is the sum of the component scores and can range from 0 to 21, with higher results indicating lower sleep quality. The empirically determined cut-off value is five, which allows for the distinction between good and bad sleep quality. All subjects with scores higher than five were excluded from the study.

The MEQ is one of the most widely used subjective tools to differentiate chronotypes. The questionnaire consists of nineteen questions to assess the subjects' preference in planning and timing of daytime activities and whether they are more likely to be highly alert in the morning or in the evening. The MEQ scores are grouped into five categories: definite evening type, moderate evening type, neither type, moderate morning type and definite morning type. There is evidence that the quality of the marital relationship is higher in partners with similar sleep/wake patterns than in mismatched couples (de Waterman and Kerkhof 1998). In our sample only two pairs were moderately mismatched (moderate evening type with moderate morning type).

During the investigation subjects were asked to spend at least ten nights together and ten separately. Sleep condition, subjective sleep assessment, sleep times, sexual activity and dreams were recorded in a sleep log based on a standardised sleep questionnaire (Self assessment scale for sleep and awakening quality: SSA; Saletu et al. 1987). Subjective sleep and awakening quality was the combined score of awakening quality (e.g. feeling refreshed after getting up) and sleep quality measures (e.g. deep and sound sleep).

In addition, the sleep-wake patterns were monitored by wrist-worn actigraphs (Cambridge Neurotechnology, Cambridge, UK). Data analysis was based on the *Actiwatch Sleep Analysis* software (Version 3.31, Cambridge Neurotechnology, Cambridge, UK). The parameter chosen for analysis of a condition ('sleeping alone' versus 'pair-sleep') and sex-grouping (female, male) base was sleep efficiency (= proportion of sleep during the period of staying in bed). In order to assess the effects of disruptive movements of one partner on another the sleep fragmentation index was used. This refers to transitions from inactive to active periods that are probably not associated with sleep. Although fragmentation is a contributing parameter to sleep efficiency, and is often strongly correlated with it, the two parameters have a different database and can be interpreted differently.

The pairs produced a total pair-sleep dataset of 249 pair or solitary nights for the females and a similar number for the males. Of these, 123 were pair nights, 126 were solitary nights. Forty-four of the pair-sleep nights were without sexual contact and fifty nine with sexual contact. The ratio of pair-sleep to solitary nights was the same for each pair.

A permutation repeated measure ANOVA (within-subject ANOVA) for unequal sample sizes was used for statistical analysis. This employed repeated measurements of the same individual over time.

Results and a Number of Open Questions

Sharing sleeping space with the opposite sex had pronounced negative effects on sleep in women, as documented by objective (actigraphic) measurements of sleep efficiency and subjective assessments of sleep and awakening quality (sleep log). Sexual contact mitigated the negative subjective impression without changing the objective results. Men sleeping alone reported a lower sleep quality than women sleeping alone. Their subjective sleep quality was raised to the same level as reported by females sleeping alone by the presence of the other sex with or without sexual contact. Also actigraphic results documented that – unlike in females – in male sleep efficiency was not reduced by the presence of their partners and their movements. Only during nights with sexual activity, also in males, sleep efficiency was significantly reduced. Thus, there was a gender difference in the reaction to the partner. We also monitored data on dream recall, as reported in the sleep logs. Interestingly, there were also gender differences. The frequency of male dream recall doubled from the 'sleep alone' to the 'pair-sleep with sexual contact' condition. In females, it decreased by 35% from the 'sleep alone' to the 'pair-sleep' condition.

The study unequivocally documented that pair-sleep is more disturbing for females than males. This fact has many implications. It must be considered when examining gender differences in the frequency of sleep disorders, effects of sleep deprivation on sleep physiology, metabolism, stress management and cognition (cf. Bennington & Heller 1995; Maquet 2001). It raises the question of whether prolonged partnerships with pair-sleep exasperate or even cause gender differences in sleep disorders and their related health complications. Or, on the other hand, whether some individuals or pairs might be better able to cope with the pre-programmed sleep disturbance associated with the partnership and thus be more 'compatible' as a pair (cf. also de Waterman & Kerkhof 1994).

The contribution represents both a novel approach and a novel interpretation of data associated with the effects of sleep environment on sleep quality. Our original intention was to demonstrate the positive effects of partnership on sleep, but over the course of the study and some twenty heterosexual couples that were investigated, exactly the opposite turned out to be true, especially for women. An advantage of our results as compared with those of previous studies on partner effects on sleep structure (e.g. Monroe 1969; Pankhurst and Horne 1994; Meadows et al. 2005), is that they were obtained within a 'field design', with participants in their own homes and beds, with partners that regularly sleep either alone or together, with occasional sexual contact.

The conclusion of the study was that females are disturbed by male presence and males on the other hand, feel quite 'happy' about the presence of a female in bed. The results suggest considering why gender differences occur. Are they a result of biological differences between the sexes or socio-culturally induced differences in environmental sensitivity associated with gender? Males seem to react to pair-sleep as if it were a collective or group sleep situation and sleep better. This is a biological explanation. The implicit idea is that sleep is safer and more secure in this environment. Anyhow, this should also apply to women. If it does, it has to be assumed that the bed structure, the closeness to the partner and the duration of the contact produce the discrepancy between the biological need for security and the documented loss of sleep quality. Women appear to be more reactive to the presence and movement of another individual in their bed. Biologist would have it that this is a logical consequence of the maternal role in human reproduction associated with infant sleep and development. They would ascribe the difference to sex dimorphism in brain structure and perceptive capacities. Most other researchers would assume that the effects are a product of upbringing and the difference in the culturally determined and modulated gender roles. Our opinion is that both of these explanations have merit and that the relative components of biological differences and socio-culturally induced reaction types differ among individuals.

These results should make the general public aware of the fact that pair-sleep at night is just a recent cultural development and, although common today at least in Western-type societies, it may impair physical or mental health by disrupting sleep. This is a poorly documented issue in sleep analysis. There appears to be a gender difference in the reaction. Here, studies on homosexual pairs are necessary for comparison. Sleep environment is not usually considered a focus in research on sleep or biological rhythms. The results presented here open up a potential impact of the sexual environment on sleep quality and demonstrate that the impact may be more pronounced for females (see also Hislop et al. 2005). It is known that prolonged sleep disruption can have negative effects on metabolism, immune function and stress responses. So the bottom line would be to determine:

© Frank & Timme   Verlag für wissenschaftliche Literatur

- whether pair-sleep is recommendable for couples
- whether the structure of the bed or mattress could mitigate negative effects on sleep quality
- whether couples may eventually habituate to one another to lessen the disruption or whether some individuals or couples are better suited for pair-sleep
- whether female sensitivity to the male during sleep is affected by her cycle phase or the use of progestin-based contraceptives
- and finally, whether the male-induced sleep disruptions contribute to higher frequencies of sleep disorders in women along with their related psychological and physiological consequences.

Acknowledgements

We wish to thank Stanislav Katina (University of Vienna), Georg Gittler (University of Vienna), Josef Zeitlhofer (Medical University of Vienna), Marietta Keckeis, Pia Pilvi, Susanna Rainesto, Ivo Machatschke and Elisabeth Graetzhofer for their help in the project.

Bibliography

AUBERT, VILHELM AND HARRISON WHITE (1959a) 'Sleep: A Sociological Interpretation I', *Acta Sociologica* 4(2): 46–54.

AUBERT, VILHELM AND HARRISON WHITE (1959b) 'Sleep: A Sociological Interpretation II', *Acta Sociologica* 4(3): 1–16.

BENINGTON, JOEL H. AND CRAIG C. HELLER (1995) 'Restoration of Brain Energy as the Function of Sleep', *Progress in Neurobiology* 45: 347–360.

BRUNT, LODEWIJK (2003) 'Between Day and Night: Urban Time Schedules in Bombay and Other Cities', BRIGITTE STEGER AND LODEWIJK BRUNT (eds) *Night-time and Sleep in Asia and the West: Exploring the Dark Side of Life.* London: RoutledgeCurzon, 171–191.

BUYSSE, DANIEL, CHARLES REYNOLDS III, TIMOTHY MONK, S.R. BERMANN, DAVID KUPFER (1989) 'The Pittsburgh Sleep Quality Index: A New Instrument for Psychiatric Practice and Research', *Psychiatry Research* 28: 193–213.

DITTAMI, JOHN, MARIETTA KECKEIS, IVO MACHATSCHKE, STANISLAV KATINA, JOSEF ZEITLHOFER, GERHARD KLOESCH (2007) 'Sex Differences in the Reactions to Sleeping in Pairs versus Sleeping Alone in Humans', *Sleep and Biological Rhythms* 5: 271–276.

EKIRCH, ROGER A. (2001) 'Sleep we Have Lost: Pre-Industrial Slumber in the British Isles', *American Historical Review* 106: 343–386.

GLEICHMANN, PETER R. (1980) 'Einige Soziale Wandlungen des Schlafes' (A Few Social Transformations of Sleep), *Zeitschrift für Soziologie* 9(3): 236–250.

HERLIHY, DAVID (1995) 'Biology and History: the Triumph of Monogamy', *Journal of Interdisciplinary History* 25(4): 571–583.

HICKS, ROBERT A. AND ROBERT J. PELLEGRINI (1991) 'The Changing Sleep Habits of College Students', *Perceptual and Motor Skills* 72: 1106.

HISLOP, JENNY AND SARA ARBER (2003) 'Sleep as a Social Act: A Window on Gender Roles and Relationships', SARA ARBER, K. DAVIDSON AND J. GINN (eds) *Gender and Ageing: Changing Roles and Relationships.* Maidenhead: McGraw Hill/Open University Press, 186–205.

HISLOP, JENNY, SARA ARBER, ROBERT MEADOWS AND SUSAN VENN (2005) 'Narratives of the Night: The Use of Audio Diaries in Researching Sleep', *Sociological Research Online* 10(4): 1–16.

HORNE, JIM AND CARL O. OESTBERG (1976) 'A Self-Assessment Questionnaire to Determine Morningness-Eveningness in Human Circadian Rhythms', *International Journal of Chronobiology* 4(1): 97–110.

IGLOWSTEIN, IVO, OSKAR G. JENNI, LUCIANO MOLINARI AND REMO H. LARGO (2003) 'Sleep Duration from Infancy to Adolescence: Reference Values and Generational Trends', *Pediatrics* 111: 302–307.

JENNI, OSKAR G. AND BONNI B. O'CONNOR (2005) 'Children's Sleep: An Interplay Between Culture and Biology', *Pediatrics* 115(1): 204–216.

KLOESCH, GERHARD, GEORG GRUBER, PETER ANDERER AND BERND SALETU (2001) 'Activity Monitoring in Sleep Research, Medicine and Psychopharmacology', *Wiener Klinische Wochenschrift* 113(7–8): 288–295.

KLOESCH, GERHARD, JOHN DITTAMI AND JOSEF ZEITLHOFER (2008) *Ein Bett für zwei* (A bed for two). München: Herbig Verlag.

LI YI (2003) 'Discourse of Mid-Day Napping: A Political Windsock in Contemporary China', BRIGITTE STEGER AND LODEWIJK BRUNT (eds) *Night-time and Sleep in Asia and the West: Exploring the Dark Side of Life.* London: RoutledgeCurzon, 45–65.

MAQUET, PIERRE (2001) 'The Role of Sleep in Learning and Memory', *Science* 294: 1048–1052.

MEADOWS, ROBERT (2005) 'The Negotiated Night: An Embodied Conceptual Framework for the Sociological Study of Sleep', *The Sociological Review* 53(2): 240–254.

MEADOWS, ROBERT, SUSAN VENN, JENNY HISLOP, NEIL STANLEY AND SARA ARBER (2005) 'Investigating Couples' Sleep: An Evaluation of Actigraphic Analysis Techniques', *Journal of Sleep Research* 14: 377–386.

MONROE, LAWRENCE J. (1969) 'Transient Changes in EEG Sleep Patterns of Married Good Sleepers: The Effects of Altering Sleeping Arrangement', *Psychophysiology* 6(3): 330–337.

PANKHURST, FRANCESCA P. AND JIM A. HORNE (1994) 'The Influence of Bed Partners on Movement during Sleep', *Sleep* 17(4): 308–315.

ROSENBLATT, PAUL C. (2006) *Two in a Bed. The Social System of Couple Bed Sharing.* State University of New York Press.

SALETU, BERND, PETER WESSELY, JOSEF GRÜNBERGER AND MARIA SCHULTES (1987) 'Erste klinische Erfahrungen mit einem neuen schlafanstoßenden Benzodiazepin, Cinolazepam mittels eines Selbstbeurteilungsbogens für Schlaf- und Aufwachqualität (SSA)' (First clinical experiences with the new sleep-inducing benzodiazepine 'cinolazepam' utilising the self-assessment scale for sleep and awakening quality (SSA)), *Neuropsychiatrie* 1: 169–176.

SCHWARTZ, BARRY (1970) 'Notes on the Sociology of Sleep', *Sociological Quarterly* 11(Fall): 485–499.

STEGER, BRIGITTE (2004) *(Keine) Zeit zum Schlafen? Kulturhistorische und sozialanthropologische Erkundungen japanischer Schlafgewohnheiten* ((No) time to sleep? A study on sleep in Japan from the perspective of social and cultural sciences). Münster: LIT.

TAYLOR, BRIAN (1993) 'Unconsciousness and Society: The Sociology of Sleep', *International Journal of Politics, Culture and Society* 6(3): 463–471.

WATERMAN, ALFRED L. DE AND GERARD KERKHOF (1994) 'Sleep-Wake Patterns of Partners', *Aviation, Space and Environmental Medicine* 65(7): 654–660.

WILLIAMS, SIMON (2005) *Sleep and Society. Sociological Ventures into the (Un)known,* London: Routledge.

WITTMANN, MARC, JENNY DINICH, MARTHA MERROW, TILL ROENNEBERG (2007) 'Social Jetlag: Mis-Alignment of Biological and Social Time', *Chronobiology International* 23 (1–2): 497–509.

WORTHMAN, CAROL M. AND MELISSA K. MELBY (2002) 'Toward a Comparative Developmental Ecology of Human Sleep', MARY A. CARSKADON (ed.) *Adolescent Sleep Patterns: Biological, Social, and Psychological Influences.* Cambridge: Cambridge University Press, 69–117.

WULFF, KATHARINA AND RENATE SIEGMUND (2000) 'Circadian and Ultradian Time Patterns in Human Behaviour: Part 1: Activity Monitoring of Families from Prepartum to Postpartum', *Biological Rhythm Research* 31 (5): 581–602.

Conflicting Sleep Demands:
Parents and Young People in UK Households

SUSAN VENN AND SARA ARBER

Introduction

The sociology of sleep has evolved since the early observations by Vilhelm Aubert and Harrison White (1959) of the influence of social and family structures on sleep patterns. Indeed, sociologists have now firmly established their presence within the topic, both by studying sleep as a physiological phenomenon influenced by social factors (Hislop and Arber 2003a; Steger and Brunt 2003; Meadows et al. 2005) and, as a result of recent empirical investigations, providing a 'window' onto the negotiation of family and social roles (Hislop and Arber 2003b; Williams 2005; Venn et al. 2008). The sociology of sleep is pushing the boundaries further by expanding existing links with other disciplines to explore diverse, but equally important and neglected areas of sleep, such as the meanings and experiences of poor sleep for older people (SomnIA 2007) to better understand this so-called 'period of remission' (Schwartz 1973: 19).

In the UK and US, the link between sleep and health is now firmly established, with ever-increasing numbers of self-help websites suggesting advice on how to achieve the 'correct' amount of sleep at the 'appropriate' time, largely through improving 'sleep hygiene' (National Sleep Foundation 2007; British Snoring and Sleep Association 2007). The aim of encouraging sleep hygiene is to facilitate the achievement of seven to eight hours of uninterrupted sleep. Sleep hygiene has, however, not always held the same medical significance. In nineteenth- and twentieth-century Holland, for example, sleep hygiene had a different cultural and moral connotation (cf. Montijn in this volume). Montijn reflects on how people were urged to maintain cleanliness in their sleeping environment. Failure to comply was seen as bad housekeeping, a sign of bad morals and was ultimately linked to the defining of a person's status. No such moral implication accompanies sleep hygiene advice today in the UK and US.

Instead we are urged to maintain strict routines of going to bed and getting up at the same time every day, and cutting out coffee, and alcohol (Horrocks and Pounder 2006; Smith and Battagel 2004). However, current 'sleep-hygiene' advice and clinical research on the physiology of sleep does not take into account how social roles influence night-time sleep. Even if a woman takes advice on how to achieve a good night's sleep by reducing her caffeine intake, her sleep may still be interrupted by her concerns as a mother for a crying child, or as a daughter worrying about a sick and elderly parent (see also Bianchera and Arber in this volume).

Sleep is influenced by many aspects of an individual's social circumstances, including their gender role, other social roles, health and changes that occur across the life course, such as having children, or returning to paid employment (Hislop and Arber 2003a). For adults sharing a bed, the quality of one individual's sleep is likely to be affected by the presence of the other. If one bed-partner has problems sleeping, this is likely to contribute to the disruption of their partner's sleep (Strawbridge et al. 2004; Beninati et al. 1999). Therefore the manner in which couples negotiate sleep and potential interruptions to sleep is important for physical and emotional well-being.

Existing clinical research on the sleep of pre-adolescent and adolescent children, and young adults over the last 20 years has recognised that young people are subject to physiological alterations to their circadian rhythms, leading them to go to bed later and get up later (Taylor et al. 2005; Wolfson and Carskadon 1998). Recognition of the effects these changing circadian rhythms have on young peoples' sleep patterns and daytime performance has even resulted in delays to school start times in one state in the US (Wahlstrom et al. 1999). However, there has only recently been recognition that social pressures on young people can also result in 'counterproductive' sleep patterns (Graham 2000). Research has suggested that whilst having televisions, computers and game consoles in young people's bedrooms significantly delays bedtimes and so reduces sleep quantity, the ubiquitous use of mobile phones has a major impact on the quantity and overall quality of their sleep (Van den Bulck 2003, 2004). Of cultural interest here is the contrast with the perception of mobile phones in terms of sleep in Japan that Kaji's research on 'knick knacks' demonstrates (Kaji 2007). Mobile phones are perceived in Japan as items that assist sleep, rather than interrupt it, by offering reassurance and security.

The development of a sociology of sleep has led to awareness that sleep is not only dynamic in terms of physiological processes, but also in terms of social processes, particularly in households with children. The structure of households has undergone change, with recent trends indicating that families are becoming more complex, often comprising children, siblings, step-siblings and other household members (Ermisch and Murphy 2006). Additionally, more young people are remaining in the family home until their twenties and thirties, delaying the transition to adulthood (Irwin 2000). It is therefore important to contextualise household sleeping arrangements in the UK in terms of the increasing trend towards teenagers and young adults living at home for longer periods.

Recent research has demonstrated how one marker of transition into adulthood that young people make, is the establishment of their own bedroom as private space, a space which is not accessible to parents, but a space from which they can continue with their social networks (Hodkinson and Lincoln 2008; Moran-Ellis and Venn 2007). As young people delay leaving home, or, as is increasingly occurring, periodically return as young adults to live at home, their expectations of increased autonomy, as reflected in a lack of rules governing bedtimes, have consequences for all members of the household (Mitchell and Gee 1996).

In this chapter we show how the complexity of everyday household living arrangements influences how and when we sleep, and even where we sleep. Sleeping for members of a household containing teenagers and young adults is at best subject to occasional interruptions, and at worst, frequent and chaotic disruptions. However, whilst our focus is on interruptions to the suggested appropriate requirement of seven to eight hours' sleep at night, we also demonstrate that for both parents and young people household noise and activity may sometimes have a positive effect on sleep, by affording a sense of security, comfort and reassurance.

The aims of this chapter, therefore, are to examine how parents and young people interact with each other's sleeping space and sleep time. First, by exploring the influence on parents' sleep of having teenagers and young adults living in the home. Second, to look at sleep from the perspective of young people, by examining how parents, other household members and technologies, such as mobile phones, influence their sleep. Finally, the positive aspects of sleep interruption expressed by both parents and young people will be examined, as, for example, when entering each others' sleeping space and time provides peace of mind and security, and can, in some instances, facilitate sleep.

Methods

Two sets of data will be drawn on to address the aims of this chapter. One set relates to parents' perspectives on sleep within the family context and the other takes the perspective of young people themselves. Firstly, semi-structured in-depth interviews were conducted with 15 couples (aged 20–59) with children over the age of 13 years. Of these 15 couples, 8 had at least one child living at home and the children of the remaining 7 couples' had left home permanently, or returned home intermittently. All the interviews were audio tape recorded and took place in the couples' own home by the first named author or female co-researchers and a male colleague[1], and lasted approximately one and a half hours. A first joint interview with the couple explored topics such as the quality, quantity and nature of sleep, with particular emphasis placed on sleep expectations and how these compared with their sleep reality. Questions were also asked about external influences on the quality of couples' sleep, such as children, caring for other members of the family, pets and so on, as well as physiological influences on the quality of sleep, such as the need to go to the toilet, snoring and pain. Each partner was then asked to record details about the quantity and quality of their sleep onto an audio tape recorder on a daily basis for one week. This audio 'sleep diary' has proved successful in previous research (Hislop and Arber 2003a; Hislop et al. 2005).

A follow up audio-recorded interview took place approximately 4–6 weeks later with each partner being interviewed separately, but concurrently. This follow-up individual interview explored in more detail issues that arose during the couple interview and by each partner in their audio sleep diaries. The interviewer and partner being interviewed were gender matched, because it was felt that same sex interviews would invoke a greater rapport between the respondent and the interviewer and provide a greater depth of data.

The second set of data comprised two focus groups held by the first named author, one with 5 boys and one with 5 girls, aged 13/14, to obtain information about sleep/wake preferences and influences on their sleep. The focus group members were then asked to keep an audio sleep diary for one week. A further 10 young people aged 13–18 were also asked to keep sleep diaries for one week, and were able to choose whether to write, tape record or e-mail their entries, or to post them on a sleep web log (blog). The young people were also

----

1   Robert Meadows and Vicky Vaughan, Department of Sociology, University of Surrey, Guildford,
     Jenny Hislop, Research Institute for Life Course Studies, Keele University, Keele.

© Frank & Timme   Verlag für wissenschaftliche Literatur

asked to make a photographic record of their sleeping environment and to reflect on their reasons for choosing these photographs, including what their photographs meant to them in terms of sleep. All interviews and focus groups were recorded and transcribed and all names used in this chapter are pseudonyms[2].

(Non) Sleeping Parents – Worries, Uncertainty and Everyday Disturbances from Older Children

This section explores how living in a household with teenage children and young adults influences the sleep of parents, particularly by examining the impact of the different sleep-wake patterns and schedules of their children. When comparing how their children interrupted their sleep when they were younger, to the present, the majority of couples commented that their sleep was more disturbed now by worrying about where their older children were at night or in the early hours of the morning. In contrast, when their children were younger, the most common interruptions to sleep resulted from physical needs, such as hunger, illness, or bad dreams, and as such were easy and quick to deal with. Gender is significant here, in that couples reported that mothers experienced greater sleep disturbance when their children were younger, because they were more likely than their partners to get up and deal with their children's' needs in the night. However, both parents were likely to have sleep interrupted by their older children.

Whilst for parents in general, and mothers in particular, the physical demands made on them at night declined as their children grew up, worry and concerns about their children did not. Recognising that the mothers were more likely to get up and go to their children when they were younger, they were also more likely to acknowledge the change in the type of sleep interruptions resulting from teenagers or young adult children. Mothers commented that they were considerably more deprived of sleep now that their children were approaching adulthood than when they were younger:

---

2   Ethical approval was obtained from the University of Surrey Ethics Committee. Written informed consent was obtained from each participant in advance, and consent was also obtained from the parents of those under 16 years.

Interviewer: Which was more difficult to deal with, when they were coming in late as teenagers or when they were small children?

Justin: I think teenagers.

Interviewer: Okay, why do you think that?

Jane: Only because of the uncertainty. I think it is the uncertainty side of things really. Not knowing, I mean it is the other things, it is not just like when they were coming in. It is like who are they out with? Who is driving? But when they were sort of safely tucked up in bed, just going and reassuring them, if they were disturbed, didn't really disturb my sleep. (Son and daughter, 21 and 19 years, couple interview)

At least with younger children, there was no ambiguity about their safety, and sleep could be quickly restored in between night-time interruptions by small children. The uncertainty of not knowing where their older children were, when they were coming in, or whether they were safe meant that sleep, for some parents, was considerably more disturbed:

Claire: If they do go out, supposing our daughter is in town, we will go to bed and we will be fast asleep. But then we will wake up early in the morning, and I will tiptoe into her room, and if she is not there, then we will panic, but she is usually there, and I will come back again so … we do worry indirectly. (Son and daughter, 20 and 18 years, couple interview)

Even when their children had left home and peaceful nights returned, parents often mentioned that when their children returned for visits home, the disturbance to their sleep returned with them:

Emma: They come back occasionally and disrupt our life, and then disappear again. They breeze their way through the contents of the fridge and freezer and invite all their friends to doss on our living room floor, and then will disappear again! (Two children, 23 and 24 years, couple interview)

© Frank & Timme   Verlag für wissenschaftliche Literatur

Sleep disturbance because of worrying did not even cease once children had left home. However, in line with expected gender behaviour, it was women who were more likely to undertake 'emotion work' or 'sentient activity' on behalf of their family (cf. Hochschild 1983; Mason 1996; McKie et al. 1999), and to be undertaking socially attentive roles (Williams 2002). Sentient activity, or invisible thinking, as suggested by Jennifer Mason (1996), is undertaken largely by women, and involves thinking about, anticipating and interpreting the needs of their partners, their children and other family members. This is not activity manifest in a physical way, as implied by 'caring for', and involving labour such as preparing food or doing household chores (Finch and Groves 1983), but rather in accord with Davidson's (2001) concept of 'unselfishness' in that it is unseen and empathetic. However, whilst this sentient activity is undertaken in relation to their family members' well-being, it is sometimes to the detriment of women's own well-being, and their own personal needs. It was, therefore, mostly mothers who reported waking at night worrying about the welfare of their children who had problems:

> Diane: Well, I am a worrier [at night] about different sorts of things. Our daughter has a money problem, that sort of really stresses me out. (Two married daughters aged 32 and 29 years, couple interview)

But it was not necessary for their children to have problems to cause parents to lie awake worrying in the night, as one mother reported, even though her children were happily settled and living away from home, the 'habit' of worrying at night continued:

> Theresa: I had a habit, I think, where I used to lie in bed and review the day and I did that quite often. I think mums do that quite often, you know, after a day and I began to get into that habit … that could keep me going and I have been trying to break myself of that habit. (Three children, 23, 27 and 29 years, couple interview)

Whilst worrying in general about their children's whereabouts at night was mentioned by all parents, driving or being driven was one of the most commonly identified night-time concerns, as reflected in the quote by Jane earlier.

Concern for family security is often remarked upon as being stereotypically gendered, in that men fulfil the role of family protector, and women support their partner in this role (Fox and Murry 2000). Women are likely to build up social relationships within their community to support their family (Ribbens 2004), whereas men's approach to family safety orients towards their own family and household. Whilst children are young, safely tucked up in bed at night, and, as was characteristic of the couples in this chapter, mothers were largely responsible for night-time care, the fathers did not need to fulfil the role of protector.

However, it is suggested that the men's perceived role as family protector, allied with an increased commitment to their children's welfare as mothers return to work, led the fathers to become engaged to a greater extent in thinking about and anticipating their older children's safety. It is not to say that the mothers were not similarly engaged, but that it was also undertaken by their partners:

> *Colin: Is he [son] lying in a river drunk? Which he did once on his eighteenth birthday … He got into the river and out of the river but after that we thought, well, next time he might just fall into the river and then die you know … (Son and daughter, 20 and 18 years, couple interview).*

Whilst the data do indicate that both parents were concerned for the safety of their children whilst out at night, maternal concerns were expressed in terms of 'worrying' in general, whereas fathers more specifically commented on worries about their children driving, or being driven. This is illustrated in the following quotation where the mother is concerned about whether her daughter has enough food and money, whereas her husband focuses on his daughter's driving:

> *Jane: I mean I quite worry about her now in London, don't I? [to husband]. So is she all right, if she has got money. If she has got enough food and things like that. I suppose more than when they were little.*

> *Justin: Who is driving? When they got to the point, when they could either drive themselves or someone was driving them. Will they have an accident? It was more what might have happened out there, that didn't bring them safely home. (Son and daughter 21 and 19 years, couple interview)*

Again, it was fathers who were more likely to remark on how they could not sleep until they knew their teenage children were home safely and in bed, and that they would often lie awake listening for them to return safely:

> Roger: *They are out to ridiculous hours in the morning and so you go to sleep at 10.30 or whatever, but always on your mind, they are both driving and subconsciously I suppose … and if you wake up at say at 12, and you think they are not in yet. So, of course, it starts [worrying for their safety] … (Son and daughter, aged 17 and 20 years, couple interview)*

A frequent concern was not just that their children were driving, but the potential danger of being driven by someone else:

> Brian: *I was always more frightened about him being in other people's cars [at night]. (Son, aged 18 years, couple interview)*

Gender of the child was also a factor in worrying about driving. There was an expectation that young men would be more reckless in cars, whereas young women would be safer drivers, but more vulnerable to the reckless driving of others:

> Kate: *It gives me palpitations now thinking about it. The first time [our daughter] went off in the car [at night] on her own and you are just, your mind does work overtime doesn't it, about what could happen. I couldn't relax until she was in, and then in some ways it is worse with a young lad [son] because they are speed merchants. I know the statistics of them having accidents and getting killed, and you just really worry. You think all the mates are in their car and geeing them up to go faster and … (Daughter aged 22 years, son aged 20 years, couple interview)*

Laying awake at night, or waking up in the night worrying about the safety, whereabouts and well-being of their young adult children was often spoken of by parents, and to some extent, whilst not anticipated, was accepted. However, what was more difficult to accept were interruptions from their children's night time activities in the house, such as cooking, making noise and playing music, which adversely affected their sleep.

Parents commented that their children were not always quiet when returning home after being out at night. Bringing friends back, and raiding the fridge for food were intrusions mentioned by several parents as interrupting their own sleep. Sometimes they were already awake listening for their children, but at other times they were woken up by them:

> Penny: But yes, you would wait to hear them come in or you would hear them come in and at times, well they made toast didn't they when they had been out, and I could smell burnt toast upstairs. Again I can't relax, because I knew they would be cooking or doing whatever and they did. They were watching a video and left the toast in the toaster and it smelt the house out. (Son aged 34 years, daughter aged 29 years, couple interview)

One father recorded over his one week's audio sleep diary how his children regularly came in and woke him up to let him know they were in and to have a 'chat':

> Roger:
> Friday 13th February: ... woken again by [our son] at around twelve o'clock coming in, had a chat for about five minutes and the same again, at around one o'clock by [our daughter] ...
>
> Saturday 14th February: [Our son] came in around 2.30, we talked for about five minutes ...
>
> Sunday 15th February: ... [Daughter] came in around, I would say, twelve o'clock, woke up and we had a chat then, dozed back off, [our son] then came in around two. Had a chat with [son] ...
>
> Monday 16th February: Kids came in at various times, obviously they woke us up. (Son and daughter aged 17 and 20 years, audio sleep diary)

Other, less frequent, interruptions to parents' sleep included children telephoning for help when a car had broken down, or calls from distressed young people when relationships had ended.

© Frank & Timme   Verlag für wissenschaftliche Literatur

The difference, however, for the parents of older children, is that whilst they expected to be woken up in the night when they have young children, it was not expected that this would continue as their children grew up. Intrusions and awakenings in the night for parents continue beyond the interruptions of babies and toddlers needing care in the night, in spite of their own expectations that their children's increased independence would lessen this. For both mothers and fathers, worrying about the location of their teenage and young adult children was frequently commented on as being significantly more disruptive in terms of a good night's sleep than when their children were younger. In line with recognised gender behaviour, women's sleep was interrupted by worrying about their children during the night, even after their children had grown up, left home and had children of their own. Fathers also worried about their children during the night, but they worried considerably more now their children were older, than when they were infants. Fears for the safety of their young adult children, particularly when driving or being driven, were the main cause of worrying at night by fathers, reflecting their concerns for their children's safety, and situating themselves within a perceived role of 'family protector'.

Among these couples, an inherent part of living in a household with more than one generation were everyday (night) disturbances, particularly young people being noisy when they came in after a night out, bringing friends with them, and, occasionally, telephone calls from young people in difficulties. One might question why parents did not apply rules about being quiet at night to their older children or require them to return home before their parents' typical bed time. However, it is recognised that teenagers are under pressure to grow up faster (Elkind 2001), and therefore expect to have more control over decisions, such as when to come home at night. Young adults living at home are often working full time and have autonomy in their daily lives, therefore parental control is less feasible and household routines may sometimes conflict. This situation has become exacerbated as young adults now remain living in the family home for longer because of extended education, difficulty obtaining their own housing and later age of marriage or cohabiting.

When exploring the meaning of sleep for couples, and for young people in households, it is important to take account of the changing demographic circumstances that are characteristic of modern family life. Although the majority of people in the UK currently live in what is officially called a 'family household', this type of living arrangement is declining (Ermisch and Murphy

2006). The trend is for a greater range of types of households, for example, the number of reconstituted families is increasing, and often comprise children who are the natural offspring of both parents, as well as children who are the offspring of one of the parents (Ermisch and Murphy 2006). Whilst the implications for these changes are far-reaching in terms of, for example, housing needs and social security, it is also important to be aware of the implications for how families negotiate and manage day-to-day living, and potential day-to-day conflicts. One example of this is the management or (non)negotiation of sleep within complex family structures where siblings, step-siblings, step-parents, boy/girl friends and other family members all seek to establish control over their sleep space and time. The second part of this chapter discusses how the sleep of young people is affected by both their situation within the household, and their own choice of sleep pattern and place.

(Non)Sleeping Teenagers and Young Adults – Worries, Uncertainty and Everyday Disturbances

The transitions that children make socially as they move into adolescence and young adulthood are accompanied by a transition into a different sleep pattern, and both types of transition can potentially cause conflict with parents and other members of their household. Teenagers and young people may also experience sleep difficulties, sometimes caused by friends and family, but sometimes because of their desire to maintain social networks into the night. However, it is important to recognise how their situation within the hierarchy of the household plays a part in constructing their sleep.

Worry and stress are well documented for adults in terms of their impact on sleep and as a recognised cause of sleep interruptions (Hall et al. 2000; Ackerstedt et al. 2002). However, significantly less attention has been paid to the influence of worry and stress on young people's sleep, except that stress and depression are more often reported as being the effect, rather than the cause, of sleep disturbance (Kirmil-Gray et al. 1984). It is expected and accepted that during the progression of the life course there will be times when sleep is interrupted by worries and concerns, for example about family, work and health (Hislop and Arber 2003b), but usually only once adulthood has been reached.

When focusing on teenagers and young adults, the primary emphasis of sleep researchers has been upon the technologies that invade their personal bedroom space in terms of causing sleep disturbance (Van den Bulck 2003, 2004). They are not, it seems, expected to be worrying about life events at this stage of their life course. However, the young people discussed in this chapter did refer to worry on many occasions, and reflected on how it delayed them getting to sleep, and affected the quality of their sleep:

> Camilla: Sleep refused to come easily last night, so I read until 1.20 a.m., when my mind finally started to quieten down. Despite the fact it was my maths exam the next day, all I could think about was the chemistry exam that I wouldn't be taking until Thursday. I was up at 7.20 a.m., quite prepared to go back to sleep for another hour, or even longer. (E-mail sleep diary, 15 years)

Whilst recognising that the data was collected during a period of public examinations for some of the young people, this was not the only cause of worry, and even those not undertaking exams often commented on how 'worries' disturbed their sleep:

> Lawrence: I have lots of things that I worry about, so often I stay up thinking, because I can't go to sleep very easily. (Focus group, 14 years)

> David: I feel really bad, we are moving soon away to near Birmingham, it's a bit upsetting really, it's going to be quite hard for me. (Focus group, 14 years)

Worries and concerns are clearly present in the narratives of young people about their sleep, with exam stress, family worries and worries about the future frequently expressed. These, however, were not the most frequently expressed causes of broken sleep, most commonly discussed was the influence of other members of the household and friends.

Friends, siblings, step-siblings, parents and even friends of siblings were commonly blamed for interrupting or cutting short teenage and young adults' sleep. Interruption to sleep at night was most often caused by older siblings and their friends when they came in late, and morning disturbances were by younger siblings or parents preparing for the day ahead:

Susan: Mum woke me up by accident when she was cleaning in the kitchen, that was at about 6 a.m.

Susan: They [brother and friend] come in late at night and raid the fridge, and put on the icemaker – it's so noisy! (Sleep blog, 16 years)

Rachel: I lay in bed until 12 [midnight] trying to fall asleep. It didn't really work though because my brother and his girlfriend were in the kitchen giggling and making loads of noise. (Sleep blog, 15 years)

Siblings were also the cause of interrupted sleep when their schedules intruded on the young persons' morning routine. For some of the young people, there was an expectation that they would accompany siblings to their morning activities:

Lawrence: Hi, it's Saturday morning, sorry, really, really exhausted, but have to get up because [brother] has acting class, and [sister] has ballet, so we are going into Guildford, it's 7.30 a.m. right now. (Audio sleep diary, 14 years)

Even absent parents can be a reason for curtailed or disturbed sleep, either because of the possibility of being able to stay up late, or as in the second extract, a sense of insecurity when parents are away:

Jenny: I went to bed very late last night, about midnight because my parents were out, so my sister and I were watching TV. (Sleep blog, 15 years)

Elizabeth: My parents being away also accounts for me waking up in the night, as I get quite worried due to an overactive imagination!!!! (Written sleep diary, 17 years)

The complex construction of modern families and households has the potential to complicate sleeping arrangements, for example when parents are divorced or separated and children have two sleeping places – one with their father and one with their mother. Household sleep can be further complicated when there are step-siblings, and decisions have to be made about who sleeps

© Frank & Timme   Verlag für wissenschaftliche Literatur

where, when and with whom. The children, whose parents had separated, explained how complex their household arrangements were:

> *Emily: I'm 14, my house is very confusing, it will take ages to describe. I have my dad and a step mum, and I've got a brother and sister who are little. I go there every weekend, and then I've got my mum and my step dad, my older brother and two little sisters in the house I live in. My older brother is 17, and there is a 7 year old, a 6 year old, a 5 year old and another 5 year old. (Focus group, 14 years)*

The impact on young peoples' sleep because of these dual living circumstances varied, from having to get up very early to comply with visiting rights, to actually improving sleep because of the bedroom arrangements:

> *Lawrence: On Tuesday, I get up at 6 o'clock and go to my dad's in the morning. I go to sleep again when I get there to make the most of the time, until 7. (Focus group, 14 years)*

> *Emily: When I'm at my dad's, my younger step-sister prods me and pokes me until I get up. (Focus group, 14 years)*

> *David: In my dad's house we have got shutters and it makes it really easy to sleep because it is quite dark and you don't know what time of day it is, no natural daylight. (Focus group, 14 years)*

Among young people with separated parents, or step parents sleep is therefore complex, as their bedrooms and bedtimes can differ according to where they are sleeping and who else is sharing the room with them. As such, young people have to adapt their sleep needs to their different sleeping environments.

Another factor is that for young people, their shift in circadian rhythm complicates the pattern of everyday life in that their night into day transition is somewhat later than that of adults, and their sleeping patterns may leave them vulnerable to interrupted and curtailed sleep. What are seen as 'normal' daily activities for adults, such as employment, often take place in the sleep time of young people, and can therefore be problematic for young people.

Some of the young people had part-time jobs, ranging from babysitting and early-morning paper rounds to working in a newsagent, which impacted on the amount of sleep they obtained, both by postponing bedtime and by cutting sleep short in the morning. Babysitting younger siblings or as paid babysitters brought a perceived responsibility to remain awake, whilst in charge of younger children:

> *Jenny: I have babysitting today until 10.30 p.m., … I can't go to sleep on the job, so I will probably sit down and do some homework revision. (Audio sleep diary, 15 years)*

And *very* early morning waking to start a job influenced sleep quality, as well as bed and wake time:

> *Joshua: Well, last night I went to bed at 9 o'clock, because I had to get up at 4 in the morning to go to work [at newsagents], so because of that I didn't get to sleep as well, because it was on my mind I guess. (Audio sleep diary, 17 years)*

For the younger teenagers, there was often a clash between the sleep they perceived their bodies 'needed' and the other demands on their time, such as school:

> *Jane: Today was the first day back at school, so I had to wake up at 7.10 a.m.. Though I don't think I was really awake until about 10 a.m.! (Sleep blog, 13 years)*

Family members and friends influenced young peoples' sleep, as did other demands on their time such as paid employment and going to school, which young people had little control over. Nevertheless, at other times, when they did have control, they often chose to subjugate their sleep to maintaining interaction with social networks via their mobile phones.

In line with other research on the sleep practices of adolescents (Wolfson and Carskadon 1998; Fredriksen et al. 2004), the young people in this research stayed up later than they believed they should, read until the early hours of the morning and, in particular, maintained contact with friends via mobile phones, even after turning out the light to go to sleep. The use of mobile phones amongst teenagers and young people has been well documented with the emphasis on how mobile phones mediate their social relationships and

© Frank & Timme   Verlag für wissenschaftliche Literatur

disrupt sleep (Taylor and Harper 2001; Williams and Williams 2005). For the young people in this chapter, their social relationships continued after returning home from school, with many using their mobile phones to communicate with friends until late at night, first thing in the morning, and even during the night.

Texting friends and receiving texts, rather than speaking on the phone, was the most common form of interaction at night with phones left on 'just in case' a message was received. There was a perceived need to be available at all times to communicate with friends and checking mobile phones for messages was often the first action upon awakening, even before getting out of bed, in case someone had contacted them during the night. Maintaining social contacts, even with friends they would be seeing at school or college that day, was important and often continued during the night:

> Helen: It [mobile phone] wakes me up, but I like to leave it on in case someone does call me really early in the morning, so I would know. (Focus group, 13 years)

The perception that a mobile phone is useful in the bedroom 'in case' resonates with Kaji's (2007) findings, where respondents to her survey reported they felt re-assured by having their mobile phones close to them whilst sleeping 'in case' of an emergency. Kaji's adult respondents saw the mobile phone as a knick knack to facilitate sleep, not only in terms of reassurance, but also as an alarm clock or a low light. However, for the teenagers in this chapter, a mobile phone in the bedroom was only perceived as a means of communication, even if it could potentially disturb their sleep.

Intrusions into young people's sleep can be varied and frequent, but can also be self-induced, reflecting the transition from young child with monitored and regulated sleep, to autonomous young adult in charge of their own bed and sleep time. These young people reflected the current cultural norm that on the one hand, the bedroom is their own private space and not subject to unannounced intrusions by parents or other family members, but on the other hand, is also a place for continuing social contacts with friends, irrespective of the time of day or night.

Controlling the Night Time, Returning to 'Peaceful' Sleep?

For teenagers and young people the negotiation of flexible bed times and sleep times are key components in making the transition to adulthood. Gaining control over their private night-time space is important for young people as part of this transition (Williams 2005; Moran-Ellis and Venn 2007). However, as Williams (2005) suggests, whilst sleep is more 'pliable' and 'plastic' for older children, there is still an element of parental monitoring and watchfulness which continues whilst sleep takes place within the household. Additionally, the private night-time space of young people is often shared with, or invaded by, other members of the household, such as younger or older siblings or step-siblings, as discussed above.

The younger teenagers did comment on their negotiations with parents about when to go to bed and/or sleep to demonstrate they were attempting to take control of their own sleep space and time. However, achieving this autonomy often resulted in young people pushing the boundaries of the sleep window into ever decreasing amounts as they chose other activities over sleep:

> *John: I go up about half 9 to 10, and then watch TV until I get tired, and fall asleep.*

> *Interviewer: And is that your chosen time or is that the time you are asked to go to bed?*

> *John: I discussed it with my mum.*

> *Paul: Yes, we discussed it. (Focus group, 13/14 years)*

Once they have gone to the bedroom, the decision of when to go to sleep is their own. Technologies are recognised by parents as disrupting their teenage children's sleep, but are also accepted as part of the transition to early adulthood. The young person's decisions as to how much mobile phones, CD players and televisions intrude on their sleep are all part of this transition. One couple commented they were aware that their child has autonomy in her bedroom about when she chooses to watch television, when to turn it off, and even what she chooses to watch:

© Frank & Timme   Verlag für wissenschaftliche Literatur

Adam: But now, as long as we don't know what she is watching she watches it [TV]. … but you do catch the flicker as we go to bed, or we turn the hall light off …

Anne: Her room is opposite ours, so you can tell whether she has got a light on.

Adam: You can see the telly through the crack of her door, can't you. Like 'Footballers Wives', she shouldn't be watching that, you know. You can't keep them in cotton wool for ever, can you? (Two daughters, aged 13 and 15 years)

For parents, control was expressed more simply, in that freedom from interruption, freedom from worries and freedom to go to sleep when one chooses were their 'ideal' sleep criteria.

Martin: I think she [wife] likes the idea of being able to go to bed and go to sleep in her own time without anybody there disturbing her. (Two daughters aged 31 and 33 years)

Diane: I am trying to learn [to adjust to not having children]. I think mums do that quite often, you know … because I rather like the peace of, you know of having bed time to myself. (Two daughters aged 29 and 32 years)

In the end, of course, for parents peaceful, restful sleep without interruptions, is all dependent on their children's well-being, or as one respondent put it, sleep was ultimately not important 'as long as they (children) were alright' (Penny). Interrupted sleep, interestingly, was not always seen negatively, some interruptions were seen as positive and reassuring, by both parents and young people.

Sleep, Noise and Reassurance

This final section attempts to redress the balance away from the negative implications of interrupted sleep. Both parents and young people also referred to sleep disruptions that were positive and that brought about a feeling of comfort and security. This was particularly evident in the young people's photographic depictions of objects that resonated with their sleep.

Something as seemingly banal as a squeaky floorboard was seen as reassuring, and was captured in a photograph by one of the young people:

> Camilla: This is a wobbly floorboard just outside my bedroom door. Whenever you sleep upstairs you can always hear people walking in the hallway because of it, which is very reassuring. (15 years, caption to photograph)

Both parents and young people, whilst recognising that their sleep is interrupted, and/or controlled by other household members, also acknowledged the reassurance afforded them by the proximity of other members of their household. Young people were sometimes reassured by parents being watchful and monitoring their whereabouts, and parents were reassured by the presence of young people (even if they were noisy), in that their presence afforded a sense of 'completeness':

> Theresa: … when they are all home [the children], when they are visiting, and they are all at home, you sleep very well. It is wonderful to have them home. You get that feeling that you have got them all there again, and they are all well and healthy. It definitely makes a difference to a mother. (Two boys and a girl, aged 30, 27 and 23 years, individual interview)

> Wendy: I prefer it if they [parents] wait up for me. I like to say goodnight to them before I go to bed. It makes me feel more comfortable and safer. (Focus group, 14 years)

Conclusion

Parents of young children have access to advice about how to get children to sleep, how to keep them asleep, and how to manage on very little sleep. Parents of teenagers and young adult children, however, are not privy to any such advice – indeed the parents discussed in this chapter were surprised by the way their older, seemingly more independent, children continued to keep them awake, and in some instances interrupted their sleep even more than when they were young.

Worries about their children's whereabouts, and their safety were often expressed, by both parents, but fathers in particular were conscious that they were more often wakeful because of concerns for their young adult children, than when they were babies or toddlers. Driving, or being driven, were the most commonly raised issues by parents when they discussed worrying about their children at night, and fathers were more susceptible to sleep disruption by this concern. Noise and door slamming also contributed to parental sleep disturbance, and occasionally also phone calls from young people in need of help.

In terms of the construction of young peoples' sleep, this was rather more complex, in that their sleep was potentially vulnerable to interruptions by parents, siblings, friends, step-siblings' and so on. The increasing autonomy over *bed* time that young people negotiated with their parents, also led to a delay in *sleep* time, when they chose to do other activities in their bedroom rather than sleep. Demands of their daytime activities, such as jobs and school also meant they were awakening sooner than most of them would have liked. The combination of interacting with social networks, usually via mobile phones, worries and their frequently phase-delayed sleep cycle, left many of the young adult children talking of being 'totally exhausted', 'very, very tired', and even 'depressed'.

It is clear that living and sleeping within a household can leave parents and children susceptible to interrupted or shortened sleep. Yet at the same time, sleep can be aided, and feelings of safety re-assured by the presence of other household members and the everyday noises they make during the night. Looking at sleep within a household context affords many opportunities to explore the (non)negotiation between parents, children, step-children, step-parents and friends in terms of defining a time and place to sleep. Additionally, the conflict and resolution that surrounds this negotiation provides a valuable opportunity to explore how relationships in general are played out in families. Future research would benefit from looking more closely at sleep through matched parent/child dyads to explore further how the power balance within families continues to shift as young people have more say in household decisions, especially in light of the increasing number of young adult children remaining living at home for extended periods.

In this chapter, we have sought to follow a similar path to that of Ben-Ari in this volume and Moran-Ellis and Venn (2007) in exploring the interactions between parents and their children through the initiation, duration and cessation processes of sleep. However, by focusing on teenagers and young adults, the complexities surrounding familial negotiations within complex household structures is more starkly brought into view. This chapter has demonstrated how discussions in families surrounding who should sleep, when and where are influenced firstly, by changes that have been taking place in the UK to family composition, and secondly, through the negotiation for increased autonomy by young people as they make the transition into adult-hood and beyond.

Acknowledgements

The authors are grateful for funding from the Centre for Research on Ageing and Gender (CRAG), University of Surrey, Guildford and the ESRC under grant RES-000-23-0268 'Negotiating sleep: gender, age and social relationships among couples'. We would also like to thank colleagues Jenny Hislop and Rob Meadows for assistance with data collection, and Rob for his helpful suggestions and comments.

References

ACKERSTEDT, TORBJÖRN, A.KNUTSSON, P. WESTERHOLM, THEORELL TÖRES, L. AL-FREDSSON AND GÖRAN KECKLUND (2002) 'Sleep Disturbances, Work Stress and Work Hours: a Cross-Sectional Study', *Journal of Psychosomatic Research* 53(3): 741–748.

AUBERT, VILHELM, AND HARRISON WHITE (1959) 'Sleep: A Sociological Interpretation. II', *Acta Sociologica* 4(3): 1–16.

BENINATI, W., C.D. HARRIS, D.L. HEROLD AND J.W. SHEPARD JR. (1999) 'The Effect of Snoring and Obstructive Sleep Apnea on the Sleep Quality of Bed Partners', *Mayo Clinic Proceedings* 74(10): 955–958.

BRITISH SNORING AND SLEEP APNOEA ASSOCIATION. http://www.britishsnoring.co.uk (accessed October 2007).

BULCK, JAN VAN DEN (2003) 'Text Messaging as a Cause of Sleep Interruption in Ado-lescents, Evidence from a Cross-sectional Study', *Journal of Sleep Research* 12: 263.

BULCK, JAN VAN DEN (2004) 'Television Viewing, Computer Game Playing, and Internet Use and Self-reported Time to Bed and Time out of Bed in Secondary-school Children', *Sleep* 27: 101–104.

DAVIDSON, KATE (2001) 'Late Life Widowhood, Selfishness and New Partnership Choices: a Gendered Perspective', *Ageing and Society* 21: 297–317.

ELKIND, DAVID (2001) *The Hurried Child: Growing Up too Fast too Soon.* 3rd ed. Reading, MA: Addison-Wesley.

ERMISCH, JOHN AND MIKE MURPHY (2006) 'ESRC Seminar Series – Mapping the Public Policy Landscape: Changing Household and Family Structures and Complex Living Arrangements', 18 May 2006, London.
http://www.esrc.ac.uk/ESRCInfoCentre/Images/ESRC_household_tcm6-15384.pdf.

FINCH, JANET AND DULCIE GROVES (1983) *A Labour of Love: Women, Work and Caring.* London: Routledge and Kegan Paul.

FOX, G.L. AND V.M. MURRY (2000) 'Gender and Families: Feminist Perspectives and Family Research', *Journal of Marriage and the Family* 62: 1160–1172.

FREDRIKSEN, K., J. RHODES, R. REDDY AND N. WAY (2004) 'Sleepless in Chicago: Tracking the Effects of Adolescent Sleep Loss During the Middle School Years', *Child Development* 74(1): 84–95.

GRAHAM, M.G. (2000) 'Sleep Needs, Patterns and Difficulties of Adolescents. Summary of a Workshop', Commission on Behavioral and Social Sciences and Education (CBASSE). Washington DC: The National Academies Press.

HALL, M., D.J. BUYSSE, P.D. NOWELL, E.A. NOFZINGER, P. HOUCK, C.F. REYNOLDS AND D.J. KUPFER (2000) 'Symptoms of Stress and Depression as Correlates of Sleep in Primary Insomnia', *Psychosomatic Medicine* 62: 227–230.

HISLOP, JENNY AND SARA ARBER (2003a) 'Sleepers Wake! The Gendered Nature of Sleep Disruption Among Mid-Life Women', *Sociology* 37(4): 695–711.

HISLOP, JENNY AND SARA ARBER (2003b) 'Sleep as a Social Act: A Window on Gender Roles and Relationships', SARA ARBER, K. DAVIDSON AND J. GINN (eds) *Gender & Ageing: Changing Roles and Relationships.* Maidenhead: McGraw Hill/Open University Press, 186–205.

HISLOP, JENNY, SARA ARBER, ROBERT MEADOWS AND SUSAN VENN (2005) 'Narratives of the Night: The Use of Audio Diaries in Researching Sleep', *Sociological Research Online.* http://www.socresonline.org.uk/10/4/hislop.html (accessed October 2007).

HISLOP, JENNY (2007) 'A Bed of Roses or a Bed of Thorns? Negotiating the Couple Relationship Through Sleep', *Sociological Research Online.*
http://www.socresonline.org.uk/12/5/2.html (accessed October 2007).

HOCHSCHILD, ARLIE (1983) *The Managed Heart.* Berkeley: University of California Press.

HODKINSON, PAUL AND SIAN LINCOLN (2008) 'Online Journals as Virtual Bedrooms? Young People, Identity and Personal Space', *YOUNG – Nordic Journal of Youth Research* 16(1): 27–46.

HORROCKS, N. AND R. POUNDER (2006) 'Working the Night Shift: Preparation, Survival and Recovery', Royal College of Physicians of London Guide. Suffolk: The Lavenham Group.

IRWIN, SARAH (2000) 'Patterns of Change in Family and Household Structure and Resourcing: An Overview', Workshop Paper: Statistics and Theories for Understanding Social Change, ESRC Research Group on Care, Values and the Future of Welfare, University of Leeds.

KAJI, MEGUMI (2007) 'Knick knacks for Sleeping (*nemuri komono*) in Contemporary Japan', Paper presented at the Workshop New Directions in the Social and Cultural Study of Sleep, University of Vienna.

KIRMIL-GRAY, K., J.R. EAGLESTON, E. GIBSON AND C.E. THORESEN (1984) 'Sleep Disturbance in Adolescents: Sleep Quality, Sleep Habits, Beliefs about Sleep, and Daytime Functioning', *Journal of Youth and Adolescence* 13(5): 375–384.

MASON, JENNIFER (1996) 'Gender, Care and Sensibility in Family and Kin Relationships', J. HOLLAND AND L. ADKINS (eds) *Sex, Sensibility and the Gendered Body*. Basingstoke: MacMillan, 15–36.

MCKIE, LINDA, SOPHIA BOWLBY AND SUSAN GREGORY (1999) 'Connecting Gender, Power and the Household', L. MCKIE, S. BOWLBY AND S. GREGORY (eds) *Gender, Power and the Household*. Basingstoke: MacMillan, 3–21.

MEADOWS, ROBERT, SUSAN VENN, JENNY HISLOP, NEIL STANLEY AND SARA ARBER (2005) 'Investigating Couples' Sleep: An Evaluation of Actigraphic Analysis Techniques', *Journal of Sleep Research* 14(4): 377–386.

MITCHELL, B.A. AND E.M. GEE (1996) '"Boomerang Kids" and Midlife Parental Marital Satisfaction', *Family Relations* 45(4): 442–448.

MORAN-ELLIS, JO AND SUSAN VENN (2007) 'The Sleeping Lives of Children and Teenagers: Night-worlds and Arenas of Action', *Sociological Research Online*. http://www.socresonline.org.uk/12/5/9.html (accessed October 2007).

NATIONAL SLEEP FOUNDATION http://www.sleepfoundation.org (accessed October 2007).

RIBBENS, JANE (1994) *Mothers and Their Children: A Feminist Sociology of Childrearing*. London: Sage.

SCHWARTZ, BARRY (1973) 'Notes on the Sociology of Sleep', ARNOLD BIRENBAUM AND EDWARD SAGARIN (eds) *People in Places: The Sociology of the Familiar*. London: Nelson and Sons, 28–34.

SMITH, A.M. AND J.M. BATTAGEL (2004) 'Non-apneic Snoring and the Orthodontist: The Effectiveness of Mandibular Advancement Splints', *Journal of Orthodontistry* 31(2): 115–123.

SOMNIA. http://www.somnia.surrey.ac.uk 2007 (accessed October 2007).

STEGER, BRIGITTE AND LODEWIJK BRUNT (2003 eds) *Night-time and Sleep in Asia and the West: Exploring the Dark Side of Life*. London: RoutledgeCurzon.

STRAWBRIDGE, W.J., S.J. SHEMA AND R.E. ROBERTS (2004) 'Impact of Spouse Sleep Problems on Partners', *Sleep*, 27(3): 527–531.

TAYLOR, A.S. AND R. HARPER (2001) 'The Gift of the Gab? A Design Oriented Sociology of Young People's Use of 'mobilZe!'', *Computer Supported Cooperative Work (CSCW)* 12(3): 267–296.

TAYLOR, D.J., O.G. JENNI, C. ACEBO AND MARY CARSKADON (2005) 'Sleep Tendency During Extended Wakefulness: Insights into Adolescent Sleep Regulation', *Journal of Sleep Research* 14(3): 239–244.

VENN, SUSAN, SARA ARBER, ROBERT MEADOWS, JENNY HISLOP (2008) 'The Fourth Shift: Exploring the Gendered Nature of Sleep Disruption among Couples with Children' *British Journal of Sociology* 59(1): 79–98.

WAHLSTROM, KARLA (1999) *Adolescent Sleep Needs and School Starting Times.* Minneapolis, MN: Phi Delta Kappa International.

WILLIAMS, CLARE (2002) *Mothers, Young People and Chronic Illness*, Aldershot: Ashgate Press.

WILLIAMS, SIMON (2005) *Sleep and Society: Sociological Ventures into the (Un)known.* Abingdon: Routledge.

WILLIAMS, STEPHEN AND LINDA WILLIAMS (2005) 'Space Invaders: The Negotiation of Teenage Boundaries Through the Mobile Phone', *The Sociological Review* 53(2): 314–331.

WOLFSON, A.R. AND MARY CARSKADON (1998) 'Sleep Schedules and Daytime Functioning in Adolescents', *Child Development* 69(4): 875–887.

Women's Sleep in Italy: The Influence of Caregiving Roles

EMANUELA BIANCHERA AND SARA ARBER

Introduction

This chapter examines sleep of women in Northern Italy. In-depth qualitative interviews with 40 women aged between 40 and 80 years enabled examination of the intimate aspects of sleep and how these are related to the social and family context of Italian women.

The aim of this chapter is to examine the meanings that Italian women attach to sleep, and their perceptions of one of the key factors that influence their sleep. The dominant theme that emerged from the interviews as influencing women's sleep was their caregiving roles, although the interview guide was not specifically designed to examine caregiving. For this reason, the chapter focuses on how Italian women's caregiving roles shape their sleep patterns and definitions of their sleep quality. Italy provides an important case study for examining the ways that caregiving roles structure women's sleep because of the fragmented welfare provision for both childcare and eldercare. The particular intensity of family connections in Italy and close intergenerational exchanges of informal care puts into sharp relief how caring delineates the extent and continuity of women's sleep, highlighting how family roles and relationships interact and intersect with sleep.

The chapter first provides a brief review of research on women's sleep, which hitherto has primarily focused on sleep in the UK. We then provide a review of care provision, family culture and the Italian welfare state. After outlining our methodological approach, we present data on women's understandings and meanings of sleep, before examining how Italian women's caregiving roles impact on their sleep at various stages through their life course.

Sleep, Women and Family Caregiving

We spend approximately a third of our lives asleep, and getting sufficient sleep is fundamental to most aspects of our waking lives. Yet surprisingly, despite the increased interest of sociologists in researching everyday lives, there has been little interest in studying sleep as part of everyday/night life. Sleep is embedded in the social context of everyday life, yet we know little about sleep in family contexts. Sleep provides a window onto understanding how gender is played out in relationships between partners, parental-child relationships, and other caring relationships. Through a close examination of discourses surrounding sleep, a lens is provided that brings gender roles and relationships within families into sharp relief.

The gendered aspects of sleep and sleeping have received particular attention in the UK through research conducted by the Surrey Sociology of Sleep Group (cf. Hislop and Arber 2003a, 2003b, 2004, 2006; Venn et al. 2008). This body of ongoing research has examined the meanings of sleep and the everyday world of sleep among women and couples, showing how a close analysis of sleep illuminates gender roles and gender inequalities within families. This corpus of work has produced insights into how sleep is socially patterned and the impact of social context on women's and couple's sleep. In particular it illustrates how women's gender role as carer of family well-being, both for her partner and children, subsumes her own sleep needs as being of lesser importance than the welfare and sleep needs of other family members. Venn et al. (2008) introduce the concept of the 'fourth shift' to highlight the ways in which women continue to undertake caring roles throughout the night. These night-time roles are not restricted to the direct provision of care, such as attending to the physical needs of children during the night, but also relate to women's engagement in the emotional labour of worrying about and anticipating the night-time needs of their family members.

Countless scientific sleep studies have shown that women report poorer sleep quality than men (Zhang and Wing 2006), with the dominant explanation put forward by sleep scientists linked to biological or physiological sex differences. These are usually purported to relate to innate physiological differences between men and women (Manber and Armitage 1999) or women's hormone levels, particularly oestrogen (Dzaja et al. 2005; Chen et al. 2005), as well as psychological explanations for women's poorer sleep (Lindberg et al. 1997). However, few scientific studies of sex differences in sleep consider sociological explanations (Chen et al. 2005). Sociologists can contribute to understanding women's higher reported sleep problems through qualitative research. In addition, and perhaps more importantly, sociological research on sleep can reveal hidden and implicit gender norms and bases of gender inequalities within different societies.

Previous research on how women's night-time caring roles influence their sleep has been limited to the UK, and focused on providing care for children and partners (Hislop and Arber 2003a, 2003b, 2003c; Hislop 2007; Venn 2007; Venn et al. 2008), rather than how caring for frail or elderly relatives influences women's sleep. This is surprising given the very extensive research on informal caring over the last 20 years, which has examined in detail the roles and tasks undertaken by family carers, but with little attention paid to how caregiving may influence the carer's sleep.

There has been no research on the impact of women's caregiving roles on their sleep in other societal contexts than the UK. Unlike Italy, the UK is a society with an established infrastructure of state support for the care of frail and elderly people. Italy provides a contrasting welfare state to the UK, since family caregiving has strong cultural underpinnings. In Italy, there is limited state provision for the care of older people, with consequent extensive caregiving roles falling on women, as well as a family structure in which adult children tend to remain living in the family home for longer, and a gender asymmetrical division of domestic labour. These aspects of the Italian family culture and welfare state are outlined in the next section.

Care Provision, Family Culture and the Italian Welfare State

Compared to the UK, care provided in Italy is more intense, first because of Italy's family-oriented culture, and second because of gaps in the Italian welfare system, resulting in minimal state support for care delivery and an informal familiarised care model (Naldini 2003; Saraceno 2003, 2005; Trifiletti 1999). Exchanges of family caregiving and interaction between adults and their older parents occur with greater frequency in Italy than in the Northern countries (Tomassini et al. 2004), and strong intergenerational ties are manifest through high levels of co-residence and spatial proximity (Glaser and Tomassini 2000). Grandparents often provide low-cost childcare while mothers work, and midlife women are particularly likely to provide assistance in cases of poor health and disability of their parents. This intergenerational caregiving compensates for difficulties in obtaining state-provided childcare services and the lack of domiciliary and residential care for frail elderly people in Italy (Tomassini et al. 2003).

Although since the Second World War in Italy there has been a substantial change from the extended to the nuclear family system (Balbo 2000; Bimbi 1999; Saraceno 1984), co-residence between adult children and older parents is still widespread (Gierveld and Van Tilburg 2004). Historically Italian family networks tend to be less dispersed than in Northern European countries (Hollinger and Haller 1990). Living in intergenerational proximity is normative within the Italian and Mediterranean culture. Mediterranean countries have been characterised by a strong family culture that regards the care of kin in need, whether a child, spouse or frail older person, as a private matter, and female relatives have traditionally provided the majority of the assistance required (Gori 2000). For this reason the Mediterranean welfare state has often been characterised as a 'familialistic' or a 'kinship solidarity' model (Naldini 2003; Saraceno 2005; Trifiletti 1999). This 'familiarised' welfare model is based on either an implicit or explicit delegation of responsibility for caring to family and kinship support networks, which frequently substitute for government provision (DaRoit and Sabatinelli 2005). In this context, care needs are primarily fulfilled through intergenerational solidarity between families and mainly carried out by the unpaid work of women (Naldini 2003; Saraceno 1984, 2003, 2005; DaRoit 2007). These care activities lead to low rates of women's participation in the labour market; the female employment rate in Italy in 2001 was 42 percent compared with an European Union average of 55 percent (Marenzi and Pagani 2004).

Women's employment and the Italian work-life balance is characterised by limited state-supported childcare, low economic activity rates of mothers, and a substantial role played by cross-generational solidarity (Ponzellini 2006). Aassve et al. (2005) argue that the impact of child rearing on women's well-being after childbirth in Mediterranean countries is greater than in the UK and in social democratic countries in Northern Europe. The low coverage of childcare services, and their high cost and limited opening hours mean that existing public services do not provide much assistance for combining household work with paid employment in Italy (Marenzi and Pagani 2004). There is also a lack of state policies relating to maternity benefits and allowances for parents or family-friendly working hours. A long break after childbirth is

 © Frank & Timme   Verlag für wissenschaftliche Literatur

therefore frequent, particularly among women from lower social classes or in less secure jobs (Saurel-Cubizollones et al. 1999). Only 2 percent of women who were working full time before the birth of their child were employed part-time two years after the birth, compared with 49 percent in Sweden (Gutierrez-Domenech 2003).

With regard to care for older people, state provided residential care is inadequate, and Italy has the lowest domiciliary care provision in Europe. OECD reported that in 1996 only 1 percent of people aged 65 and over in Italy were recipients of home help, compared to 5.5 percent in England, 6.5 percent in Germany and 16.6 percent in Sweden (Gori 2000). This is despite Italy having the highest proportion of older people among European countries (World Health Organization 2004). In this situation, care responsibilities for elderly relatives are mainly handled by family and kin networks (Saraceno 2005). The lack of state-provided care for older people in Italy has led to a growth in privately employed care assistants from third countries. A 'care drain' (Bettio et al. 2004) has drawn migrant female workers, mainly East European, popularly called 'badanti', literally 'minders', to provide co-resident care for disabled older relatives (Daly and Lewis 2000; DaRoit 2007; Zanatta 2004; Rothgang and Comas-Herrera 2003).

The mixed care solution developed in Italy and other Mediterranean countries has created a complex division of labour. Family carers may have to coordinate personal care work by immigrant 'minders', as well as private health providers (for medical treatment), charity and third-party support (such as for taxi-driving services, and from social associations) (Simoni and Trafiletti 2004). However, the provision of home-based elderly care through this complex web of care provision does not change the gendered division of labour between women and men. Although all family members may contribute to the assistance of frail relatives in Italy, with some men involved in elderly-spouse care, those providing care are still predominantly women.

Paoletti's Italian research (1999, 2002), based on conversational analysis, shows how linguistic categories build up and associate caregiving for elderly relatives with women, and how caring is constructed conversationally primarily as a female duty. Gender categories in Italy have strong moral connotations. For instance, where a parent needs care, 'being a daughter' is sufficient reason to become a carer. Caring tasks are recognised as gender-specific practices, therefore failing to carry out these duties is sanctionable for a woman, but this is not the case for a man (Paoletti 1999, 2002).

Methods

This chapter examines Italian women's sleep drawing on the sleeper's subjective experiences and knowledge of sleep. Given the intimate dimension of sleep and the sensitive family and emotional dynamics that are interconnected with sleep, a qualitative exploratory and interpretative approach was chosen. According to Strauss and Corbin (1998: 11) 'qualitative methods can be used to obtain intricate details about phenomena such as feelings, thought processes, and emotions that are difficult to extract or learn about through more conventional research methods'. The qualitative approach is more exploratory, and is therefore appropriate for this research, which does not aim to provide a quantitative outline of sleep quality in Italy, but an in-depth understanding of the everyday experiences of women associated with sleep. An interpretative approach to analysis has been adopted 'for the purpose of discovering concepts and relationships in raw data and then organising these into a theoretical explanatory scheme' (Strauss and Corbin 1998: 11).

In-depth audio-recorded interviews were conducted with 40 Italian women aged between 40 and 80 years, including married, single, divorced and widowed women. Women who lived within approximately 30 miles of a medium-sized town in Northern Italy were recruited through local social, educational and community organisations and via snowball sampling. They were intentionally recruited to represent varied social and economic characteristics in order to investigate women's sleep in different family contexts. Pilot work was conducted before the study to test the techniques previously used in sleep research in the UK (Hislop and Arber 2003a, 2003b), particularly to refine the interview guide for a different cultural context. Interviews were conducted between January 2006 and April 2007. The study was approved by the University of Surrey Ethics Committee.

Qualitative interviews lasting approximately one hour were conducted by the first author, and recorded with each participant's permission. The aim of the open-ended questions was to capture the cultural context influencing women's sleep, particularly the impact of women's social context, family structure, and gender roles.

To analyse the qualitative interview data, a grounded ethnographic thematic approach was chosen. This allowed concepts to emerge directly from the data. The transcripts were systematically reread to identify relevant analytic themes and examine relationships between the categories, comparing and contrasting

   © Frank & Timme   Verlag für wissenschaftliche Literatur

the findings coming from the interviews. The computer-assisted qualitative data analysis software package QSR NVivo 2.0 was used to support thematic analysis and conceptualisation. Interview transcription was in Italian, with quotations subsequently translated into English. Pseudonyms are used to protect the anonymity of respondents, with their age indicated after quotations.

It is important to note that discussion of intimate dimensions related to the topic of sleep during the interviews tended to reveal detailed life-history data. Bryman (2002) notes that in contexts such as ageing research or feminist research, which deal primarily with sensitive biographical issues, through the detailed attention of the researcher, women give new meanings to experiences, awareness, and a different perception of self.

Women's Understanding of Sleep

As Rensen (2003:107) notes, to understand sleep it is crucial to consider the 'overall logic', the perspective of the sleeper and the significance they attach to their own experience of sleep.

When asked to define a good night's sleep, women describe almost unanimously their concept of uninterrupted, unfragmented sleep, and a qualitatively deep sleep, often testified by dreams. Women identified lack of consecutiveness and continuity in sleep as the major factor defining a poor sleep quality. A bad night's sleep was generally signified the following day by the feeling of not being rested.

> *Sleeping well means falling asleep and waking up the next day, without interruption. Sleeping bad is when you wake up four, five times during the night, so that in the morning I wake up more tired than when I went to bed. (Chiara, 55)*

> *Sleeping bad means waking up frequently, sleep but feeling you did not sleep. You wake up in the morning and say 'did I sleep, did I not sleep?' having bad dreams, waking up tired. I have experienced it myself and know what it means not to sleep well. (Luisa, 67)*

I sleep well if I can sleep in a continuous way, for many hours. I sleep badly if I have my sleep interrupted, fragmented and non-consecutive.
INT: Can you give examples of interrupted sleep?
For example, if I have an emotional situation of anxiety for something that happened during the day, then my sleep is restless, I wake up frequently. Or external factors, like the child that does not feel well and wakes up. Then I have to get up and be present, and sleep does not continue relaxed as before. (Francesca, 41)

Women saw sleep as positive for their well-being, as well as for their functioning during the following day. In addition, sleep was valued as providing a time of personal space, and intimacy, in which women experienced freedom from their daily obligations, and the possibility of 'feeling themselves'.

Night for me is a moment of detachment from reality, a moment also for myself, where, in a way, I find again a time for myself. Where I do not have to do anything for anyone else, but finally be myself. Consequently it is also a moment of intimacy with myself as well as of regeneration, rest and recovery of energy. It also has this significance. (Francesca, 41)

For me, sleep is liberating, sleep is getting free from a series of fatigues of the day; therefore I don't feel it is wasted time. I feel it as a time of absolute freedom, possibility of freedom, in the real sense of the word. (Annamaria, 41)

Sleep is another kind of wake. How to say, it is another aspect of living, very rich, very intense, very vital, and for me of great support to the time when I am awake. Therefore, there is an enrichment, a reciprocal give and take between sleep and wake. (Beatrice, 52)

Some women considered that dreaming and remembering dreams was a signifier for them of a good night's sleep.

If I wake up and remember a dream then … I feel more rested, even if dreams are not beautiful. But if I remember them, it seems to me that this period of sleep has been profitable, productive. (Laura, 48)

© Frank & Timme   Verlag für wissenschaftliche Literatur

If I remember dreams in the morning it means that I slept well, even if the dreams are not nice. It means that I slept to dream. On the contrary, when I wake up and do not remember the dream I feel more tired ... (Paola, 45)

When reflecting on how sleep had changed across their life course, women identified two distinct phases divided by marriage, or alternatively by taking on caring roles for children or for other relatives. Sleep in the earlier phase of their life course was characterised as a personal space for the self, and a time of intimacy for themselves. Whereas during the second phase, sleep was seen as occupying a shared dimension, in which they lacked personal control over the quality of their own sleep. The dominant factor distinguishing sleep during the second phase was one of caring for other family members.

INT: How does sleep change when the family grows?
It changes a lot because before sleep used to be like a closed world, including just yourself. Later, as your family grows, it becomes something different: even if you wanted to close down, there's nothing you can do, there's a window open onto the lives of the others ...
Sleep no longer gives me that relaxation, that total closure of years gone by. Now it's a very different thing, it's more physical. I don't feel it's my own thing anymore, to say 'it's my own world'. To me it has always been important, because it was a world just for myself, with my own thoughts ... Now you think about the others, it's not your space anymore. (Maria, 64)

When I was a girl waking up it was worse in the sense that you say 'I have to wake up and go to work'. But it is another kind of sleep, you sleep well, without worries, you don't worry for anyone but yourself. You marry, you have a family, you start to get worried, not only for yourself but for others. You say: 'In my house I can decide my own timetables'. It's not true, because if one works you have to prepare meals at a given time, you have to wake up the child in the morning getting her ready for school, when they are little they cry at night, and also having a child is a very big responsibility, if he is well or not well. Your life changes completely, and also sleep ... There is the difference between having a family and being free. It's a totally different thing. (Renata, 64)

Although, these two phases of sleep quality may be distinguished by the birth of a child, this change in sleep quality was not always because of the onset of caring roles, but in a minority of cases related to childbirth being associated with other changes in the woman's life. For example, Francesca illustrates that she had poor sleep quality prior to her marriage and childbearing due to the worries associated with her high-powered job, which at the time caused her to lie awake at night worrying about her work. In addition, her sleep was interrupted because of the stresses and worries associated with her situation in Italy as an unmarried women in her late-thirties living alone.

> *The child is my great divide. There is a before the child and an after the child. This is, let's say, the frame. Before I used to read before sleeping; it helped me relax and quieten my mind. Now, because I am more tired, it is rare that I can read anything. Before I often had a restless sleep because of work. I used to wake up at 3, 4 in the night. So the night sleep was not continuous. Now after the first few months, when I breastfed, now the child sleeps all night and, unless she wakes me up by crying, I sleep deeply all night through until seven. So there are no phases of awakening connected to work-related worries or personal distress [...]*
> *Sleeping on your own, from an objective point of view, is ideal. But then (before marriage) I had awakenings where I thought about my condition, my life as a single woman, also that kind of worries. Now I have fewer awakenings related to internal uneasiness, but instead caused by external objective factors (children), that in the end ... let's say that sleep quality has improved because now I am able to sleep all through the night. I do not have emotional distress, so I don't have these awakenings that happened before, which previously adversely affected my sleep. (Francesca, 41)*

In general, the interviews with Italian women illustrate that their sleep can be divided into two broad phases, that as a younger single person without caring roles and responsibilities, and secondly, sleep following marriage and motherhood. For the majority of women, their narratives about the latter tended to be dominated by the ways in which their caring roles and responsibilities defined their sleep quality and duration.

During the second phase, we can distinguish the ways that sleep is influenced by two conceptually distinct aspects of family caregiving: first by the physical aspects or tasks of providing care to a child or to a frail older person during the night, and second, by the worries and anxieties associated with women's role as family care-provider. Our focus in this chapter on these two ways in which women's role may have an impact on their sleep, does not mean that other factors unrelated to caregiving do not. For some women their sleep is interrupted by worries about aspects of their lives other than caregiving, as illustrated by the quotation from Francesca above. Her sleep prior to getting married and childbearing, was adversely affected by worries associated with her stressful occupation, and by her anxieties about still being a single woman in her late thirties, where the cultural norm in Italian society is one of marriage and childbearing.

This chapter cannot do justice to an examination of all the factors that may be implicated in the quality of Italian women's sleep, therefore we focus on the theme that was dominant in our interviews, namely the ways in which women's caregiving roles have major potential for framing the timing, quality and duration of their sleep.

It is important to bear in mind that there may be qualitative differences in the perceptions of women about different types of sleep interruptions associated with caregiving. Caring for children at night can be seen in a positive way, even when it affects women's sleep, whereas providing care to elders is more likely to be seen negatively by women in terms of sleep disruption. For example,

> I have tended my mother at night, who slept in my room, as I remember. And then I assisted an elderly relative with a terminal illness for one month, my father-in-law who was dying … I can't really tell you, I can just perceive that if I sleep with a newborn child there is a certain effect, different from an elderly person … I think that if you sleep close to a newborn you feel … when I was tending my daughter, surely sleep quality was different, more pure … While sleeping close to an elderly relative can create anguish, maybe because you acknowledge that they are doing a journey which anticipates yours. (Donata, 59)

Our data illustrate how sleep quality and duration are connected with the care for the majority of midlife and older Italian women. Through care provision, sleep may lose the characteristics of a self-owned, personal space for relaxation, and become a shared dimension where the needs of the receiver of care (both physical and emotional) become central. For most women caring is a life-long experience, combining practical tending with emotional activity. Although husbands and other family members contribute to family caregiving, women predominate as carers in the UK and even more so in Italy. In the following sections, we illustrate the ways in which caregiving at different phases of the life course influences Italian women's sleep.

Sleep and Caregiving Through the Life Course

Women identify undertaking the role of carer as a turning point in the way in which they experience their sleep. In particular, the birth of a child generally acts as a borderline separating two distinctive sleeping lives. The sleep of a mother is more alert, and more sensitive to the needs of the child, is matched to the child's sleep patterns, being 'tuned in' on the child's cry, as in these examples:

> *The children have changed my sleep considerably, especially when they were little, because you kind of 'tune in' … if they just do something, speak or cry, my two sons, I hear it. It's like a frequency – you are tuned in on their cry, on their call. I think it's something related to maternal instinct, because it has never happened before. If one of the two has a problem, it is always me that goes, my husband does not hear them. (Veronica, 46)*

> *After the birth of the child, my sleep has become lighter, because evidently I am more tense, and I wake up more than once.*
> *INT: Even if the child does not call you?*
> *Eh, yes, I wake up even if she does not call me. Because I became more anxious, silly, I recognise it, like when she is ill and I am afraid she coughs … then when she feels better you are still with your ear open … (Marzia, 42)*

In some cases child-rearing in combination with heavy work commitments can be problematic. Women who are full-time housewives may have the possibility of recovering sleep lost at night during the day. Whereas working mothers reported sleep deprivation, which had consequences for their emotional and physical well-being, mostly related to the difficulty of balancing between full-time work and childcare.

In the morning I wake up very early, like at six to do the housework. At 8, I leave for work while the grandparents come and pick up the child. When I come back from work, I go and pick up the child, wash him, then prepare the dinner, then do other housework and until late in the night I cannot go to sleep. I cannot get more than five hours sleep, and I feel bad for it. [...]

Apart from the psychological aspect, I have physical disturbances, like muscular pains, weariness, tachycardia. I try to cope by taking vitamins, but it does not help. When I am really burnt out I go to my parents' place, take two days for myself and sleep. During this time, I manage the child with my mother and I can recover, so I think it is just a matter of sleep in the end. (Elisa, 41)

Women often mention a range of issues related to work-life balance that contribute to their sleep deprivation, including limited availability of part-time jobs, difficult access to nurseries, the need to turn to family networks for childcare support, and a problematic relationship with grandparents who look after their children. A successful coordination between parents and grandparents with respect to childcare seems central to the efficiency of the childcare arrangements, the serenity of the mother and the quality of her sleep. Need for child-rearing support accounts for many women choosing to live close to their family of origin. Adele, who worked shifts as a full-time obstetrician, managed to combine childcare with her special sleep needs by living on the first floor of her parent's house:

When I married and had a family, I had already decided I would stay in my parents' house, because having seen the experiences of my colleagues, who had a family with children, all those were very problematic, from an organisational point of view. You know, with children, you have to go to work, the child is ill, the baby sitter doesn't come ... So I made this choice, obviously my husband agreed, living like this, at least I am tranquil from a family point of view ... Obviously, when children are little and start crying, you know, you are the one who wakes up, before your mother. The commitment was always there, but it was shared with my parents. (Adele, 58)

For older women, looking after grandchildren or having them close by, can lead to a sense of serenity, which promotes their sleep.

Family peace is one thing that makes you relax and sleep well in every sense. The satisfaction that ... I feel an achieved woman because I have my daughter living upstairs with her family, and if I hear noise, I know it's their children and it's like I don't even hear them. If I had somebody else living upstairs I would surely be angry. Instead, being from the family I say, 'oh it's Maria (granddaughter), there it's Antonio (grandson), it's them who are playing'. (Mariangela, 70)

Having children around also reduces loneliness among older women and provides a way for them to feel active and useful. On the other hand, caring for grandchildren can be an additional commitment which adversely impacts on older women's sleep.

The close correlation between women's sleep quality and caring is particularly evident in extended families, where caregiving occurs for several family members. Although Italian families are increasingly changing from an extended to a nuclear model, the majority of interviewed women over 60, had lived for much of their life as part of an extended family household, where care for children, grandchildren, grandparents or other relatives was undertaken and shared entirely within the household. Co-residence with other family members means first of all coordination of different sleep rhythms:

The sleep has always been light, I have always heard everything, I preferred to go to bed last, otherwise the others woke me up, and I got angry because I could no longer sleep. Anyway after a while you can combine with everyone, I have had my in-laws at home until they were 95 ..., anyway I loved them too, it's always been a well-accepted thing. (Loredana, 80)

Even though many respondents had positive experiences of support and conviviality through living within an extended family care system, women undertaking household management, child rearing and more demanding elderly assistance, often experienced problems that resulted in sleep disruption:

I worked very little outside the home, but I worked at home. Demanding families, big families. I used to have my mother-in-law, father-in-law, brother-in-law, who later moved out with his family ...
When children are little, sleep is very limited. You sleep if they sleep, you sleep if they are well. Then during the day you have little time for your-

self... Then the years have passed, my father died, my father-in-law got ill. And yet we still didn't sleep, because he used to wake us up, he escaped, shouted. ... There has been the death of (brother), the illness of my husband, altogether. You sleep, because you have to make up your mind and realise that you also have to think about yourself, otherwise you won't be able to struggle with the others' suffering. But sleep changes, you sleep less. You wake up all of a sudden, because maybe you know that they don't feel well and they need you. At the very moment they call, you are already there ... you don't sleep deeply. (Luisa, 67)

This account by Luisa, for whom care had been an ongoing commitment throughout her life, illustrates how the experience of caring in an extended family is interrelated with her sleep quality.

Caring for Elderly Family Members

Providing assistance to frail elderly family members was usually seen by women as having a substantial influence on their sleep and well-being. Depending on the type of illness, extent of required support and relationship with the ill person, caring for an elderly relative can be experienced as worthwhile or stressful. Where the care is shared (with sisters, brothers, or other relatives) and the caregiving is temporary and not overpowering, women reported less effect of caring on their sleep quality ... However for some women the caregiving demands were overwhelming and expectations overcame the carer, with their physical and psychological health becoming affected. The most adverse consequences for sleep occurred during and after particular types of care provision such as: assistance during terminal illnesses; assistance during unpredictable illnesses; and assistance during long term illnesses, including night assistance.

In cases of dementia or the terminal phase of illnesses, sleep disruption often becomes frequent, unexpected and more upsetting. In these cases the lack of domiciliary welfare support in Italy becomes more evident and emerges in the accounts of women as compounding caring responsibilities at night and sleep deprivation.

My grandmother, the grandmother I had at home ... she was ill for six months with cancer, she was terminally ill ... When this thing happened, it was really very, very grave because of the lack of structures to support us with this type of illness, because her being terminally ill, no structures existed to support this kind of problem. Therefore, we found ourselves having to take her home (from hospital), and spend the nights with her ... in shifts, my mother, me, my brother when he could, because he had an extremely demanding job. Going to sleep at 4 in the morning, when she fell asleep, and waking up after an hour, one hour and a half, was a routine ...

I will tell you that this thing has lasted for about one year, after the death of my grandmother – I had a hard time falling asleep, in sleeping, in regaining a regular rhythm of sleep. I had really a hard time. Because I could still hear her – I heard her voice calling me, because she was in need, or it seemed to me that my mum would call me, because she needed help with her ... all these sorts of things. It took me a year to regain the regular rhythm of sleep. (Lina, 54)

Assistance during terminal illness, which is also connected to the distress of bereavement, may have long-term adverse effects on sleep. This often continued for long after the death of their relative, and mainly resulted in night-time awakenings, light sleep and insomnia, which was sometimes treated by sleep medication.

When women had caregiving support from family members, both practical and emotional, this gave them personal space, which could be dedicated to work or rest, and the overall caring burden was better managed, resulting in less sleep disruption.

The impact of caregiving is therefore moderated by the woman's family structure (i.e. presence of other women or available helping relatives in the family) and by socio-cultural and economic circumstances (i.e. alternative paid care is more often sought by women with higher income and more education). These issues are discussed in more detail in Bianchera and Arber (2007).

Conclusion

This chapter, based on qualitative interviews with women over the age of 40 in Northern Italy, examines women's understandings of sleep and illustrates how sleep is intrinsically inter-related with women's caring roles, showing how family care shapes sleep structure, continuity and extent.

Women's basic assumption of what represents a good night's sleep is a night of unfragmented deep sleep. This understanding changes with the transition from the status of single woman with no caring responsibilities to the status of carer for multiple family members. Women tend to distinguish between two qualitatively different meanings of sleep, attached to these two different phases: in the first phase sleep is a self-owned dimension of intimacy; in the second it is a shared dimension intimately connected with the needs of other family members. In this second phase, sleep patterns and definition are shaped through the physical and emotional aspects of caregiving. In general, negative experiences are often associated with providing care to frail elderly relatives, while more rewarding experiences are connected to child rearing. The data we have presented show how sleep in the Italian informal care system is related to the coordination and management of intergenerational care among the family network.

Caregiving in Mediterranean countries is characterised by a strong family culture, where support and mutual help within the family is socially encouraged. Assisting children and frail elderly relatives is generally regarded as a private matter, and the responsibility of the family. The fragmented welfare provision in Italy and gender segregation within families means that the major burden of domestic and caring work falls on women. Sleep problems are most likely to be found in difficult situations of care – for example, when women do not receive family or external support, or have to deal with severe assistance problems, especially when caring for elderly or disabled relatives, and may last for substantial periods after caregiving ceases.

The nature of gender-role expectations and family welfare responsibilities impacts on Italian women's sleep and well-being. Sleep is shown to be influenced by family care worries. It reflects pressures at difficult stages of the life course and varies in concert with the nature of family commitments. This does not mean that women's sleep is not affected by other factors beyond the family, such as work-related worries, other stress or environmental factors, but a consideration of these influences on sleep is outside the scope of this chapter.

This chapter has shown how family caregiving influences women's sleep, defining, helping or disrupting it. To understand sleep, it is crucial to place it in an intergenerational family context. For women, particularly in a Mediterranean context, care for family members is closely interrelated with the dynamics of sleep, with both positive and at times problematic implications.

Acknowledgements

The authors are grateful for funding from the EU Marie Curie Research Training Network on 'The biomedical and sociological effects of sleep restriction' (MCRTN-CT-2004-512362).

References

ARBER, SARA AND JAY GINN (1995a) 'Gender Differences in Informal Caring', *Health and Social Care in the Community* 3: 19–31.

ARBER, SARA AND JAY GINN (1995b eds) *Connecting Gender and Ageing*. Buckingham: Open University Press.

BALBO, LAURA (2000) 'Working and Living with Equal Opportunity', *Inchiesta* 30(127): 1–3.

BETTIO, FRANCESCA, ANNAMARIA SIMONAZZI AND PAOLA VILLA (2004) 'The "Care Drain" in the Mediterranean: Notes on the Italian Experience'. Paper presented at the 25th Conference of the International Working Party on Labour Market Segmentation, Brisbane, Australia.

BIANCHERA, EMANUELA AND SARA ARBER (2007) 'Caring and Sleep Disruption among Women in Italy', *Sociological Research Online* 12(5). http://www.socresonline.org.uk/12/5/4.html.

BRYMAN, ALAN (2002) *Biographical Research*. Buckingham: Open University Press.

CHEN YING-YEH, KAWACHI ICHIRO, S.V. SUBRAMANIAN, DOLORES ACEVEDO-GARCIA AND LEE YUE-JOE (2005) 'Can Social Factors Explain Sex Differences in Insomnia? Findings from a National Survey in Taiwan', *Journal of Epidemiology and Community Health* 59: 488–494.

DAROIT, BARBARA (2007) 'Changing Intergenerational Solidarities within Families in a Mediterranean Welfare State: Elderly Care in Italy', *Current Sociology* 55(2): 251–269.

DAROIT, BARBARA AND STEFANIA SABATINELLI (2005) 'Il modello mediterraneo di welfare tra famiglia e mercato', *Stato e Mercato* 2: 267–290.

DALY, MARY AND JANE LEWIS (2000) 'The Concept of Social Care and the Analysis of Contemporary Welfare States', *British Journal of Sociology* 51(2): 281–298.

DZAJA, ANDREA, SARA ARBER, JENNY HISLOP, MYRIAM KERKHOFS, CAROLINE KOPP, THOMAS POLLMÄCHER, PAIVI POLO-KANTOLA, DEBRA SKENE, PATRICIA STENUIT, IRENE TOBLER AND TARJA PORKKA-HEISKANEN (2005) 'Women's Sleep in Health and Disease', *Journal of Psychiatric Research* 39: 55–76.

FINCH, JANET AND DULCIE GROVES (1983) *A Labour of Love: Women, Work and Caring.* London: Routledge and Kegan Paul.

GIERVELD, JENNY DE JONG AND THEO VAN TILBURG (2004) 'Living Arrangements of Older Adults in the Netherlands and Italy: Co-residence Values and Behaviour and their Consequences for Loneliness', *Journal of Cross-Cultural Gerontology* 14(1): 1–24.

GLASER, KAREN (1997) 'The Living Arrangements of Elderly People', *Reviews in Clinical Gerontology* 7: 63–72.

GLASER, KAREN AND CECILIA TOMASSINI (2000) 'Proximity of Older Women to their Children. A Comparison between Britain and Italy', *The Gerontologist* 40: 729–737.

GORI, CRISTIANO (2000) 'Solidarity in Italy's Policies towards the Frail Elderly: A Value at Stake', *International Journal of Social Welfare* 9: 261–269.

GUTIERREZ-DOMENECH, MARIA (2003) 'Employment After Motherhood: A European Comparison', CEP Discussion Papers dp0567, Centre for Economic Performance, LSE.

HISLOP, JENNY (2007) 'A Bed of Roses or a Bed of Thorns? Negotiating the Couple Relationship through Sleep', *Sociological Research Online* 12(5). http://www.socresonline.org.uk/12/5/2.html.

HISLOP, JENNY AND SARA ARBER (2003a) 'Sleepers Awake! The Gendered Nature of Sleep Disruption among Mid-Life Women', *Sociology* 37(4): 695–711.

HISLOP, JENNY AND SARA ARBER (2003b) 'Understanding Women's Sleep Management: Beyond Medicalization-Healthicization?', *Sociology of Health and Illness* 25(7): 815–837.

HISLOP JENNY AND SARA ARBER (2003c) 'Sleep as a Social Act: A Window on Gender Roles and Relationships', SARA ARBER, KATE DAVIDSON AND JAY GINN (eds) *Gender and Ageing: Changing Roles and Relationships.* Maidenhead: Open University Press, 186–205.

HISLOP, JAY AND SARA ARBER (2006) 'Sleep, Gender and Ageing: Temporal Perspectives in the Mid-to-later Life Transition', TONI CALASANTI AND KATHLEEN SLEVIN (eds) *Age Matters: Realigning Feminist Thinking.* London: Routledge, 225–246.

HISLOP, JENNY, SARA ARBER, ROB MEADOWS AND SUE VENN (2005) 'Narratives of the Night: The Use of Audio Diaries in Researching Sleep', *Sociological Research Online* 10(4). http://www.socresolnline.org.uk/10/4/hislop.html.

HOCHSCHILD, ARLIE (1983) *The Managed Heart.* Berkeley: University of California Press.

HOCHSCHILD, ARLIE (1990) *The Second Shift: Working Patterns and the Revolution at Home.* London: Piatkus.

HOLLINGER, FRANZ AND MAX HALLER (1990) 'Kinship and Social Networks in Modern Societies: A Cross-Cultural Comparison among Seven Nations', *European Sociological Review* 6(2): 103–124.

JAMES, NICKY (1992) 'Care = Organisation + Physical Labour + Emotional Labour', *Sociology of Health and Illness* 14(4): 488–509.

LINDBERG, EVA, CHRISTER JANSON, THORARINN GISLASSON, EYTHOR BJORNSSON, JERKER HETTA, AND GUNNAR BOMAN (1997) 'Sleep Disturbances in a Young Adult Population: Can Gender Differences be Explained by Differences in Psychological Status', *Sleep* 20: 381–387.

MANBER, RACHEL AND ROSEANNE ARMITAGE (1999) 'Sex, Steroids and Sleep: A Review', *Sleep* 22: 540–555.

MARENZI, ANNA AND LAURA PAGANI (2004) 'The Labour Market Participation of "Sandwich Generation" Italian Women'. rlab.lse.ac.uk/lower/final_papers/pagani.pdf.

MASON, JENNIFER (1996) 'Gender, Care and Sensibility in Family and Kin Relationships', JANET HOLLAND AND LISA ADKINS (eds) *Sex, Sensibility and the Gendered Body*. Basingstoke: Macmillan, 15–36.

MEADOWS, ROBERT (2005) 'The "Negotiated Night": An Embodied Conceptual Framework for the Sociological Study of Sleep', *The Sociological Review* 53(2): 240–254.

NALDINI, MANUELA (2003) *The Family in the Mediterranean Welfare States*. London: Routledge.

PAOLETTI, ISABELLA (1999) 'A Half Life: Women Caregivers of Older Disabled Relatives', *Journal of Women and Aging* 11(1): 53–67.

PAOLETTI, ISABELLA (2002) 'Caring for Older People: A Gendered Practice', *Discourse & Society* 13(6): 805–817.

PARKER, ROY (1981) 'Tending and Social Policy', ELSA MATILDA GOLDBERG AND STEPHEN HATCH (eds) *A New Look at the Personal Social Services*. Discussion Paper No. 4. London: Policy Studies Institute.

PONZELLINI, ANNA (2006) 'Work-Life Balance and Industrial Relations in Italy', *European Societies* 8(2): 273–294.

RENSEN, PETER (2003) 'Sleep Without a Home: the Embedment of Sleep in the Lives of the Rough-Sleeping Homeless in Amsterdam', BRIGITTE STEGER AND LODEWJIK BRUNT (eds) *Night-Time and Sleep in Asia and the West. Exploring the Dark Side of Life*. London: RoutledgeCurzon 87–107.

ROTHGANG, HEINZ AND ADELINA COMAS-HERRERA (2003) 'The Mixed Economy of Long Term Care in England, Germany, Italy and Spain'. Paper presented at the 4th International Research Conference on Social Security 'Social Security in a Long Life Society'. Antwerp, 5–7 May 2003.

SARACENO, CHIARA (1984) 'Shifts in Public and Private Boundaries: Women as Mothers and Service Workers in Italian Daycare', *Feminist Studies* 10(1): 7–29.

SARACENO, CHIARA (2003) *Mutamenti della famiglia e politiche sociali in Italia*. Bologna: Mulino.

SARACENO, CHIARA (2005) 'Path Dependency and Change in Welfare State Reforms in the Southern European Countries', 19 December. www.sante.gouv.fr.

SAUREL-CUBIZOLLES, MARIE-JOSÈPHE, PATRIZIA ROMITO, VINCENTA ESCRIBA-AGUIR, NATHALIE LELONG, ROSA MAS PONS AND PIERRE-YVES ANCEL (1999) 'Returning to Work after Childbirth in France, Italy and Spain', *European Sociological Review* 15(2): 179–194.

SIMONI, SIMONETTA AND ROSSANA TRIFILETTI (2004) 'Caregiving in Transition in Southern Europe: Neither Complete Altruists nor Free Riders', *Social Policy and Administration* 38(6): 678–705.

TOMASSINI, CECILIA, DOUGLAS WOLF AND ROSINA ALESSANDRO (2003) 'Parental Housing Assistance and Parent Child Proximity in Italy', *Journal of Marriage and the Family* 65: 700–715.

TOMASSINI, CECILIA, GRUNDY EMILY KALOGIROU STAMATIS, TINEKE FOKKEMA, PEKKA MARTIKAINEN, MARJOLEIN BROESE VAN GROENOU AND KARISTO ANTTI (2004) 'Contacts Between Elderly Parents and their Children in Four European Countries: Current Patterns and Future Prospects', *European Journal of Ageing* 1(1): 54–63.

TRIFILETTI, ROSSANA (1999) 'Southern European Welfare Regimes and the Worsening Position of Women', *Journal of European Social Policy* 9(1): 49–64.

VENN, SUSAN (2007) 'It's Okay for a Man to Snore': The Influence of Gender on Sleep Disruption in Couples', *Sociological Research Online* 12(5). http://www.socresonline.org.uk/12/5/1.html.

VENN, SUSAN, SARA ARBER, ROBERT MEADOWS AND JENNY HISLOP (2008) 'The Fourth Shift: Exploring the Gendered Nature of Sleep Disruption in Couples with Children', *British Journal of Sociology* 59(1): 79–98.

WILCOX, SARA AND ABBY C. KING (1999) 'Sleep Complaints in Older Women Who are Family Caregivers', *Journal of Gerontology: Physiological Sciences* 54B(3): 189–198.

WILLIAMS, SIMON (2002) 'Sleep and Health: Sociological Reflections on the Dormant Society', *Health* 6(2): 173–200.

WILLIAMS, SIMON J. (2005) *Sleep and Society: Sociological Ventures into the (Un)known.* Abingdon, Oxfordshire: Routledge.

WORLD HEALTH ORGANIZATION (2004) *Better Palliative Care for Older People.* Edited by Elizabeth Davies and Irene J. Higginson. Geneva: World Health Organization.

ZANATTA, ANNA LAURA (2004) *Sintesi della ricerca su 'Lavoro di Cura, Genere, Migrazioni', Osservatorio Nazionale sulla Famiglia.* http://www.welfare.gov.it/NR/rdonlyres/ ej6axyedhjhqgpfpniq6gnxjdaayshs34zptpjlsh5fw6cx7kpsjukpqe5idv5vmkp2jz3i6ilef 5oeshpuxunfsfhb/AnnaLauraZanatta.pdf.

Sote hue log: In and Out of Sleep in India

Lodewijk Brunt

In human societies sleep is organised in varying ways. In North-West European countries, for instance, a concentrated nocturnal sleep is considered to be normal – possibly even natural. But in the Mediterranean region the phenomenon of the siesta – sleeping not only at night but also in the afternoon – is an integral part of everyday life. In other parts of the world, still different sleeping arrangements exist. In Japan, with its napping culture it is taken for granted that people take naps during the day – either privately or in public (Steger and Brunt 2003). In this contribution I deal with sleep in India and some of the ways Indian sleep is organised. Does this differ from the examples just mentioned? My effort must be rather exploratory however, because there is no anthropological or sociological tradition of sleep research in India and as far as I can tell, nobody has ever explicitly considered sleep in terms of its social arrangements.

In India sleeping is breathing. I have always been greatly impressed by the seemingly natural, easygoing way Indian people are able to sleep in any situation and under any condition. Arriving at Mumbai International Airport in the middle of the night, sleep is the first thing one is confronted with while driving downtown. Hundreds of sleeping bodies are lying on pavements or other traffic islands, seemingly undisturbed by the deafening sounds of densely packed, relentless expressways. Also, during the day sleep is abundant and everywhere to be seen. Shopkeepers, ticket sellers, taxi drivers, peddlers, doormen, hawkers, policemen are among the many people taking naps in all kinds of situations. In Mumbai whole families sleep on the floor of the crowded halls of railway stations, where trains arrive from and leave for destinations all over the gigantic subcontinent. Perhaps India has a sleep culture all of its own. But before going into Indian sleeping, I need to make a few general remarks about the country and my professional involvement with (sleep) research.

The World of India

India is a continent in itself. A surface of roughly thirty million square kilometres and a population of nearly one billion people. Boundaries – with countries like Pakistan, Tibet and China – amounting to more than 15,000 kilometres. In the North are the majestic Himalayas; in the South the Deccan Plateau flanked by fertile coastal zones. In between the hot Indian plains, dominated by the Ganges, Yamuna, and Brahmaputra, the mighty rivers which originate in the Northern mountains and flow out to the Gulf of Bengal after thousands of kilometres meandering through the densely populated land.

Although India is a predominantly agrarian society, with more than 60 percent of its population living in the countryside, cities and urbanisation are becoming more important by the day. In 1991 India had almost 25 cities with a million people or more; today, the number is more than 40. Some of the biggest cities in the world are Indian. Mumbai, Delhi and Kolkata each have between 15 and 20 million inhabitants and are growing steadily. The influence of the new urban middle classes is felt everywhere, especially on the level of federal and state policies. Enormous amounts of national and regional funds are diverted into projects for the improvement of the urban infrastructure: airports, highways, flyovers, public transportation, housing and educational institutions.

In 1991 the Indian economy was 'liberated'. The stifling *licence raj*, an inheritance of Javaharlal Nehru's socialist-inspired guided economy, was replaced by an open, capitalistic system. Economic growth has gone on its way since. On top of the pre-industrial and industrial sectors the computerised and globalised service sector and a sector of light industry and electronics came into being. In a short time this constellation led to spectacular results and the Indian 'post-industrial zone' gained a strong international reputation for electronic engineering. Today places like Bangalore are considered to be the Silicon Valleys of the East. In Mumbai and cities like Ahmedabad the industrial zones of cotton and other textiles – the famous Manchesters of the East – have lost their former prominence. After the end of the 1980s they became sites of industrial archaeology, almost overnight.

I got involved with anthropological research in India rather late in my academic career. Since the early 1990s I have been travelling to India on a regular, annual basis. Sometimes for a short trip of a few weeks, but usually for a two- or three-month stay, and occasionally for a longer period. Mumbai has been

  © Frank & Timme   Verlag für wissenschaftliche Literatur

my home most of the time, although I have travelled in every direction and have stayed for extended periods in other places as well. Even so, my personal experience of Indian society is practically limited to cities. Yet urban life and culture are as varied as anything in India. Public life in New Delhi is very different from that in Old Delhi. Both are perhaps even more different from metropolises like Mumbai or Kolkata, on the one hand, or overgrown provincial towns like Surat, Jaipur or Varanasi on the other.

I have been especially interested in the field of urban time schedules. Normally urban research is oriented towards space and spatial arrangements: Where do people live and work and how do they travel from one place to another? What's the difference between downtown and uptown? In what ways are cities connected with suburbs and the countryside? My own perspective is rather different and oriented towards the way people spend time – both individually and collectively. What are the opening and closing times of workplaces, schools and shops and are these times coordinated, correlated or not associated at all? Do harbour cities have different time schedules than administrative cities? Do urban public spaces have different characters according to the time of day or night? Hence my interest in sleep.

Indian Sleep

I never attempted to systematically study sleep as a natural, physiological phenomenon as such. In my perspective sleep is part and parcel of everyday life and should be considered in its social and cultural context. Apart from direct observation both inside and outside of people's homes and workplaces I have read extensively about sleep in classical Hindu texts but also in (auto-) biographies and contemporary Indian novels and non-fiction, mainly written or translated into English. My main object was to gain insights into the perspective on sleep and all that surrounds it. I felt this need because of my Western bias in conceiving of sleep primarily as something connected with health (see also the introduction to this volume). I looked for new angles and original points of view. I tried moreover to get some glimpses on how sleep is organised. To what extent is sleep associated with night? Are there fixed places for sleeping; fixed times; fixed rituals? To help me find my way I have also been taking photographs of 'sleepers'. I snapped random pictures of people apparently asleep in broad daylight wherever I stumbled upon them. This chapter is based on these three sources. My aim is both descriptive and exploratory, i.e. I try to outline some themes for future research, hoping that India will become a test case in the rapidly emerging sociology of sleep – similar to countries like Japan and China (cf. Steger and Brunt 2003).

First some observations. What strikes me most about Indian sleep, I think, is the absence of a clear boundary between sleeping and waking. When visiting people it is perfectly natural to conduct a conversation with some members of the household whereas others watch TV, read the newspaper, or are asleep. In cases where very small children are falling asleep they are sometimes taken to the bedroom (if there is one) and put to bed, but normally speaking this daylight sleeping occurs while other activities are taking place as well. People fall in and out of sleep just like they fall in and out of conversation. Although there are more or less generally accepted 'sleeping times', nobody seems to claim that sleeping is something one should only do in certain places and only during certain periods.

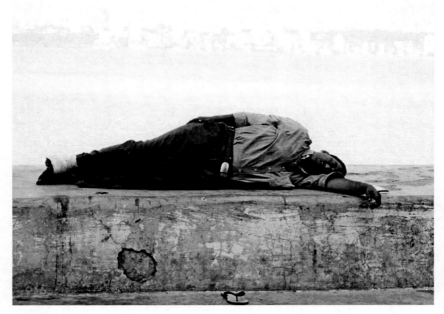

Fig. 1: Sweet dreams (photograph: Lodewijk Brunt)

 © Frank & Timme   Verlag für wissenschaftliche Literatur

Whenever I go and visit the Savants, my former neighbours in Dahisar, the northernmost suburb of Greater Mumbai, I try to behave accordingly, especially when I tell them that I'm a little tired, which is no lie after a long and hectic journey by train. Although they are well aware that I'm a bad sleeper during the day, they offer me their couch anyway. There is no harm to be done in lying down and closing one's eyes for a while. Svapna Savant even offers to massage my feet because she thinks that this will surely help me to fall asleep.

In fact the situation regarding sleep in the Savant household is rather complicated. The Savants are a family in which different sleeping habits co-exist. Svapna is a passionate sleeper who takes a nap whenever she has a moment to herself. And when she sleeps she sometimes seems to be completely in another world. She doesn't even hear the doorbell ringing when her husband or children come home. But her husband Shailesh has to be out at work all day and sleeps only at night, except for a short nap as soon as he arrives home while he waits for the food Svapna is preparing. This is during the working week because on his free Sundays – and of late he has Saturdays free as well – he's an erratic sleeper too. Sometimes, while between jobs, he is home for a prolonged period. He jokingly complains that this is not to his liking. 'All I do is eat, sleep, eat, sleep', he laughs, 'soon I will get used to this lifestyle and then I won't want to do anything else anymore'. Their two children – a son and a daughter – also take a short nap after they have been to school, but more often than not they only sleep at night. I know from other households too, how varied the sleeping habits can be depending on age, gender, work and school.

What also strikes me is the public or semi-public character of sleep. Public meaning open – in the presence of others – in contrast to sleep in Western countries, which is a personal matter, private and almost intimate. In the India I know it seems perfectly natural to sleep in public – with either intimates or complete strangers around. When my friend Arunabh Bhattacherjee and I went from Mumbai to Surat to meet the Municipal Commissioner in March 1997, we stayed at the house of a mutual friend. There was only one spare room and Arunabh and I had to share the bed. Although we hardly knew each other at the time, this was considered perfectly normal. I also remember the man who entered the waiting room at Pune train station. He was carrying a small attaché case and after he had asked for the arrival time of his train he opened it. All it contained was a kind of a blanket. He spread the cloth in the middle of the extremely crowded room and went to sleep, using his case as a headrest. In public transportation in general I'm always struck by the ease with which people seem to be able to sleep – be it in cars, buses, trains or planes. My pet theory is that Indians don't suffer from jet lag, but some informants have been trying to convince me that I'm wrong.

As a consequence of these characteristics sleep does not seem to be closely associated with specialised spaces or rooms. While walking through cities I've seen (and photographed) people sleeping on chairs, in cars, on top of cars, on bikes and rickshaws, on pavements and on station platforms, in temples, mosques, and churches, in trains and buses, on benches, on top of market stalls, in parks, in restaurants, and in theatres and cinemas. I'm not only greatly impressed by this variety of locations, but also by the conditions under which people appear to be able to sleep.

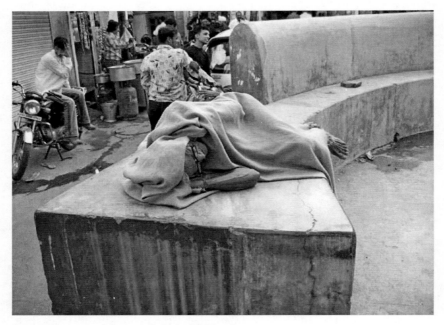

Fig. 2: Private space (photograph: Lodewijk Brunt)

I have mentioned one condition already: the crowdedness, the incredible density of the population in cities, big and small. One closely related condition is the blinding light from the blazing sun and a third is the incredible level of noise. In the Western countries that I know of, such conditions would be considered sure guarantees of a lifelong crippling insomnia, yet in India one is used to them without seeming to be bothered at all. Perhaps the opposite is true. Once I overheard a Dutch colleague of mine talking to a Dr. Desai in Surat. The topic of their conversation was Dr. Desai's mango plantation, which is situated in some distance from the greatly overcrowded city. In the middle of the plantation there lies a beautiful, spacious bungalow. 'Why don't you go and live there', my colleague asked. 'Oh, no! It's much too isolated', said Dr. Desai, adding '… it would be impossible to sleep in all that silence'. Sleeping alone, in silence, sheltered from the outside world would be a nightmare for many Indians that I know. As Salman Rushdie wrote in his famous *Midnight's Children*: '… solitude, a condition so unusual in our overcrowded country as to border on abnormality' (Rushdie 1995: 202; see also Lahiri 1999: 115).

Correspondingly it should be stipulated that although in India, just like elsewhere, night and sleep are strongly associated, nights are not exclusively reserved for that purpose. Both religious and secular ceremonies, as well as other festivities, often take place during the night, whereas many people are used to getting up very early in the morning – mostly for religious purposes as well. Dalrymple in his grandiose portrait of Delhi mentions the Holi festival in springtime. In a period of about a fortnight around this festival it seems everybody wants to get married. One can hear the deafening noise of drums and trumpets and music from Hindi films until well into the night. And before eight in the morning it starts all over again. 'Why this ceremony has to take place so early in the morning', Dalrymple (1993: 203) writes, 'has never been explained to me'. There are other periods of intensive marrying as well – all depending on priests who pronounce some days as being extremely suitable for this occasion.

My experiences in Mumbai are similar. But not only ceremonies take place at night, some working practices and forms of entertainment do too. In the late 1990s I used to travel by local train between South Mumbai and the Northern suburb of Dahisar where I lived. Often I came home after midnight and found the railway station and surroundings brimming with life. Not only where there rickshaw drivers waiting for customers, but also hawkers and shopkeepers and, of course, swarms of young boys were playing cricket loudly in the light of street lanterns. Close to my home the muslim bakery was in full swing, as was the blacksmith hammering away on the pavement in front of his workplace. I remember New Year's Eve 1997 when I stood at midnight on my little balcony watching the fireworks on neighbouring roofs. The road was being repaired in front of my compound. The work went on as if time didn't exist.

Reading About Sleep

Reading – my second source of knowledge about sleep. The literature I have studied (written or translated into English) does not explicitly deal with sleep or with related subjects as such. I'm not referring to scientific books or articles, but classical Hindu texts, novels, poetry and general non-fiction. I am interested in casual remarks about sleep and sleeping because I think such unobtrusive sources of knowledge add to the insight I have gained from direct observation. I have made notes on the concept of sleep itself. How is sleep conceived? What kind of power does sleep have? What kind of emotions are associated with sleep? Does Indian sleep have, like in many Western societies, a special connection with the night? And: How is sleep socially organised?

I am aware of the problematic nature of such a research procedure. There is no way to learn about the exact relationship with social reality, and neither is there a way to tell how 'representative' such literature is. Although I realise that this is true, I also know that much the same holds for academic literature. Both the Hindu classics and most of the contemporary novels, however, are infinitely more exciting, amusing and stimulating to read than scientific writings – that's the bonus of this approach. And in order to explore the nature of a phenomenon, I think it is permitted to use anything of potential value as long as one takes care to be modest about the results.

Let me first deal with the phenomenon of sleep itself. Both from the *Ramayana* and the *Mahabharata* – which are, according to many people, the 'holy books' of Hinduism – one gets the impression that sleeping – like eating, drinking, and working – is not just a unmanageable natural phenomenon, but something people should try control. In the best known part of the *Mahabharata*, the *Bhagavad Giitaa*, sleep is associated with laziness and indifference. According to Krishna, in a dialogue with Arjun just before the decisive battle between the Pandavas and their cousins the Kauravas, there are three basic 'personality types': harmony (*sattva*), passion (*rajas*) and dullness (*tamas*). A dull personality, which develops from ignorance, is passive and indifferent. Many low-ranking positions in society are related to dullness. Such a personality sleeps a lot. In real life people can improve their position by meditation (yoga). The first way for a yogi to reach *nirvana* is to be frugal in all things, especially sleeping. He must not sleep too much – but also not too little (*Bhagavad Giitaa* 2001: 80, 124, 125).

One of the overwhelming number of exotic characters in the Ramayana is the giant devil Kumbhakarna. The god Brahma has cursed him and as a consequence he is nearly always in a state of deep sleep. It's extremely difficult and dangerous to wake him, because after many months of sleep he is starved and he swallows everything that comes near. Sleep renders this fearsome creature unconscious and harmless. Thus, sleep might be considered as an effective punishment for antisocial behaviour (Ayyangar 1991: 1375ff). However, in general, the gods, devils and warriors in these classic stories sleep like 'normal' human beings mostly at night, but sometimes during the day as well.

One gets the impression that sleep is a force in the hands of gods or ghosts or similar forces. Not only from the 'holy texts', but also from contemporary literature. In Umrigar's *The Space Between Us*, for instance, Bhima feverishly tries to sleep, lying next to her granddaughter Maya. The girl snores softly and occasionally murmurs in her sleep. In Bhima's mind it is 'innocence' that causes Maya's childlike sleep (Umrigar 2006: 65). Elsewhere the writer mentions 'sleep monsters' that are able to kidnap a person if he is not paying attention and is sleeping during the day in public places (Umrigar 2006: 58, 59). Narayan writes about the relationship between the English teacher and his little daughter. The first thing he notices waking up is his daughter looking at him. 'Sometimes she just sat, with her elbows on the ground and her chin between her palms, gazing into my face as I lay asleep [...]. Whenever I opened my eyes in the morning, I saw her face close to mine, and her eyes scrutinising my face. I do not know what she found so fascinating there'. She just wants to watch, she says. It appears she is sometimes saying things close to his face in order to see his reaction. One day she asks him: 'What do you do when you sleep, father?' It's a question the teacher thinks cannot be answered by an adult – perhaps only by another child (Narayan 1955: 102). A similar fascination for the nature of sleep is expressed in *Sexy*, one of Lahiri's short stories. American Miranda and Indian Dev are having an affair and they meet on Saturdays. After lunch they make love and then Dev takes a nap – for exactly twelve minutes. Miranda had never before in her life seen an adult sleeping during the day. She herself never slept. After six minutes she turned to face him, sighing and stretching, testing to see if he was really sleeping. He always was (Lahiri 1999: 94).

My observation that the night is not exclusively used for sleeping finds ample confirmation in the literature as well. Gandhi's autobiography contains passages about his nocturnal existence, which was often dedicated to work or travel (Gandhi 1957: 401–403, 411). His biographer Stanley Wolpert is much more explicit and mentions Gandhi's experiments with yoga and *brahma-charya*. In his sixties he sleeps with young women from his *ashram* to master his sexuality. He is not supposed to give in to sexual inclinations but only to harbour 'motherly' feelings for them. But often it seemed necessary to communicate with the girls in the middle of the night. Manu was roused as Gandhi got up at 1.30 a.m. and started working or started dictating letters. Others have witnessed Gandhi writing his diaries during the night and Shusila spent most of her nights with him reading these diaries (Wolpert 2001: 186–187, 225–226). Kashikey (1997: 87, 159) speaks about nightly activities in Varanasi; Lahiri (1999: 115) has her Mrs Sen tell about similar situations in Bengal; Deshpande (2004: 133) and Irving (1995: 503) write accordingly about Mumbai at night, and Chughtai (2006) writes about the overlap between night and day in her youth. In the *Ramayana*, Sanjaya and the king of Hastinapura have philosophical discussions in the middle of the night (Narayan 2000: 325). At a certain moment time comes to a complete standstill after Ravan has sent away the seasons. This causes a great deal of confusion everywhere and as a consequence people sleep during the day (Narayan 2000: 99).

In the literature there are also many references to the way sleep is organised. Indian writers sometimes give the impression that afternoon sleeping is an Indian habit; they even use the word siesta, although this term must have been introduced by the British.[1] According to Mishra afternoon sleep is part and parcel of Buddhist – and perhaps Hindu – discipline and everyday life (Mishra 2004: 151). Elsewhere the same author writes about the library of the Hindu University in Varanasi. Bored students were scratching their initials into the table tops and 'some of them chose to take their siestas on long desks' (Mishra 2006: 8). Rushdie (1995), Scott (1977), Prawer Jhabvala (2000) and Lahiri (1999) use the word siesta as well. Prawer Jhabvala's story *The Temptress* is about a woman called Ma who has travelled from India to New York City and has gained some fame due to her special spiritual qualities. She spends her days thus: 'Ma went out on her excursions, cooked spicy little messes for

....

1   In Hindi there is no such word as siesta. In some English-Hindi dictionaries one is able to find the word siesta. The translation is 'descriptive'. In Raker and Shukla (1995a, 1995b) siesta is described as a 'short sleep after a midday meal'. In Hindi they say *'dopahar kii jhapkii'*, which has a somewhat more generalised meaning, i.e. 'afternoon doze'. In Hindi this translation the midday meal has disappeared. In Pathak (1939: 815) one finds 'a short sleep at midday in hot countries' as the meaning of siesta. The translation in Hindi is identical: *'garam deshom mem dopahar kii alp nidraa'*; *'alp nidraa'* meaning unimportant, insignificant, or little, sleep. In Gupta and Gupta (1999: 763) the same meaning of siesta is given, but in the Hindi expression they use is *'dopahar kaa aaraam'*, meaning 'midday rest'. They do without the hot countries and, strictly speaking, the sleep.

herself, had long afternoon naps, and watched TV' (Prawer Jhabvala 2000: 153). Chaudhuri writes about afternoons in Kolkata: a time to sleep, a time for digestion. 'Full stomachs, closed eyes' (Chaudhuri 1998: 94, 95). Crucial episodes of Irving's novel *A Son of the Circus* are situated in Mumbai's posh Duckworth Club, which for insiders is easily identifiable as the *Bombay Gym-khana* – a luxurious British colonial gentlemen's club taken over by Mumbai's bright and beautiful. In this club one finds special rooms for gentlemen taking their siestas. Afternoon naps are also written about in Narayan (1993: 42) and Gandhi (1957: 335, 336). Roy (2004: 90) mentions the forced afternoon naps of her childhood, whereas Niranjchana (2001: 85) remembers that children were often pretending to sleep.

But often in writings on Indian life sleep doesn't seem to be ordered or timed at all. In *The Tiger Ladies* Koul describes a courthouse scene. 'It had been a hot, steamy afternoon and everyone was in a state of deathlike monsoon lethargy, just a nod away from being fast asleep' (Koul 2002: 159). In his autobiography, Singh writes about his time as a lecturer in Hawaii. A couple of Japanese students used to fall asleep in his class. Singh was greatly offended by this behaviour. He took revenge by refusing to let the students pass their examinations (Singh 2002: 225). But remarkably enough, the same author doesn't seem to notice that the same kind of sleeping in his homeland India would not be considered out of place. About his period in the Indian *Rajya Sabha* (perhaps to be considered as the equivalent to the United Kingdom's House of Lords) he mentions that many Members of Parliament attended the meetings just to fart and to sleep. 'Many came because in the heat of the summer it was the coolest place to be in; the eminent Hindi novelist who for a time sat next to me was fast asleep within five minutes of taking his seat' (Singh 2002: 334). Fairly typical is the quote from *The Space Between Us*. The elderly Bhima walks home lost in her thoughts and hurts her hip when she runs into a handcart parked on the middle of the sidewalk. A young man is fast asleep on the cart and Bhima marvels at how a person is able to sleep through the noise of the surrounding crowd. She rubs her hip and asks herself whether to shake the sleeping boy to ask him to move his cart. But then she notices a bulge under his loose pyjama bottoms. 'Dirty scoundrel', she mutters, quickly averting her eyes. 'Drunken lout, lying here in the open as if he owns the city. Shameless, shameless people' (Umrigar 2006: 95). One comes across passages in which sleep is considered out of place and out of time, but there is no mention of underlying formal or informal rules or regulations.

Let me give an example of sleep rules from the Netherlands. Recently a Dutch journalist was arrested by two policemen. He had taken a rest on a bench in Amsterdam's Oosterpark and had fallen asleep. The policemen told him he was punishable on the basis of the local *Algemene Politieverordening* (General Police By-law) which forbids sleeping in public. He was given a 75-euro fine (Brummelen 2007). In India I don't know of any rules like this. The only time I have seen anything that came close was in Delhi. Just in front of the extremely crowded Delhi Central Railway Station there is a sign forbidding people, among other things, to fall asleep.

I came across the mentioning of oversleeping a number of times. The main character of Niranjchana's novel excuses herself after having slept too long. She comes down at 8 a.m. and sees her husband sitting at the kitchen table with coffee and a newspaper. She realises that she has been brought up by her mother to rise in the early morning and make coffee for all the male members of the household (Niranjchana 2001: 171). Someone has also overslept in Umrigar's novel (Umrigar 2006: 62). Only once did I notice a writer who explicitly deals with sleep disturbances and insomnia, or …? The mother of the main personage in *Midnight's Children*, is suffering from these ailments. 'Amina Sinai', writes Rushdie, 'woke up one morning with a head buzzing with insomnia and a tongue thickly coated with unslept sleep …' (1995: 65). Did Amina Sinai experience 'unslept sleep' before she woke up, in her sleep?

Bombay Times (8 February 2005) carries a remarkable article. It is about falling asleep at work. The journalist has the impression that in Mumbai insomnia is frequent. There are always deadlines to be reached, daily life in the metropolis is full of stress and people go to bed very late. It is pointed out that people have to work odd hours and night shifts and that basic sleeping patterns have been disturbed. Conclusion: 'Late nights, early mornings and stressful days – that's why Mumbai's not getting enough! Of sleep, that is!' This is the very first time I have ever seen sleep mentioned as being something of a 'problem' in India. The *Bombay Times* usually reports about the good life in big cities, about film stars and about media hype, where to eat, where to go for entertainment, and about fashion and new trends in general. It is loud and extraordinarily superficial. Could insomnia be part of a new lifestyle?[2]

---

2 Dr N. Ramakrishnan of Nithra, Institute of Sleep Sciences in Chennai, pointed out to me that especially among middle-class people, foremost women, the number of sleep complaints is quite substantial. Personally I don't know anything about this. As stated, in the literature I have been reading and in my own observations, not only in the streets but also in people's houses, I didn't come across a single case of sleep disturbance, except for one elderly lady who regularly tells me

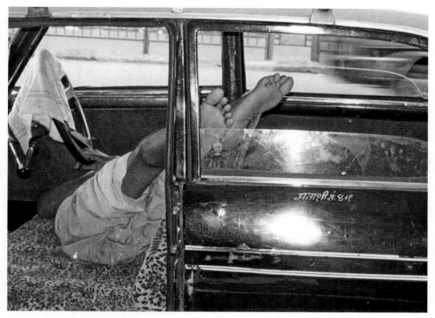

Fig. 3: Napping at the workplace (photograph: Lodewijk Brunt)

Indian Sleep: Napping Culture?

Both from my own observations and from the literature it does indeed appear that Indian sleep is omnipresent. At night, but also during the day. And not just at siesta time. Yet there doesn't seem to be much awareness about certain patterns or specific 'sleep cultures'. Even in the limited amount of books I'm quoting from, however, there are several tantalising questions and stimulating suggestions to be found. However much the sleeping climate in India might be characterised as 'liberal', sometimes people do oversleep. They seem to be breaking a rule. But what rule? Is this typical for housewives or women in general perhaps? One might think so on the basis of the above-mentioned quotes, but this is guesswork.

On the basis of my own observations I would say that there are probably gender differences in sleeping. To mention just one example: the number of

about her sleeping problems because of chronic pain.

women sleeping 'rough' – i.e. on their own, in public – seems to be small in comparison with the number of men and boys. But what about the discipline of sleep? Is that also a matter for women only? To what other questions is sleep discipline linked? Equally tantalising is the social status of sleep. In some contexts sleep seems to be considered as benevolent and positive, in other contexts sleep is a bad force, best to be avoided. One wonders about the sleep monsters as well: How general is that image? Is it something only the primitive and uneducated mind is occupied with, or is this a notion every Indian would immediately recognise? Each and every point could be the start of some interesting further research.

I find it difficult to characterise Indian sleep. Is there an Indian sleep culture different from all the other sleep cultures in the world? That doesn't seem at all plausible in view of all the social, cultural, ethnic, linguistic, and regional varieties one finds in this huge subcontinent.

Perhaps the siesta culture is a case in point. Both from my own observations and from the literature we may confidently conclude that the occurrence of afternoon naps is relatively general in India. As a concept it even has found its way into several frequently used dictionaries. Yet, it would be inappropriate to characterise India as a siesta culture as such. Why? I would say that for a siesta culture to exist some degree of societal institutionalising should be in evidence. Like for instance in the Mediterranean, where in the early afternoon not only do most people withdraw from public life, but most shops and other amenities close. Nowhere in India is this the case as far as I can tell. There may be shops and offices closing in the afternoon, but there is no general rule underlying such a practice. In India I have never experienced the silence, the empty streets and closed houses which are so typical for siesta time in some parts of France or Italy. A similar reasoning could be held for the case of India being a napping culture, i.e. a culture where people sleep whenever they feel the need and find an opportunity, irrespective of time and place. It would also be equally difficult, if not impossible, to point out general Indian institutions which are 'typical' for such a culture.

And now I arrive at my third source of information about sleep in India. As I have pointed out earlier, I have analysed a substantial amount of photographs which I – more or less at random – took of sleeping people in Indian cities. If India is a 'napping culture', I reasoned, one should find people sleeping everywhere and at any time – without them being in the least disturbed or removed from their spots. Indeed, this seems to be the case. To put it differently: (daytime) sleeping does not habitually take place at special times and/or in certain specialised spots. On the contrary, in Indian cities one sees people asleep almost everywhere in the public domain: pavements, seaside, walls, parking lots, stairs, squares, parks, benches, cars, bikes. Moreover, it is very hard to point out typical precautions or typical props people use while sleeping, nor is it easy to observe typical precautions that sleepers have taken to consider the interests of other city dwellers. On some photographs one can see people sleeping in the middle of the pavement at, say, 11 a.m. or 3 p.m. – other pedestrians have to step over them or go out of their way to get past. The sleepers seem to be at ease, they do not hide from public view, and they do not seem to get harassed or restrained in any way. As such, one could say they are the living evidence of a sleep culture in which 'anything goes'.[3]

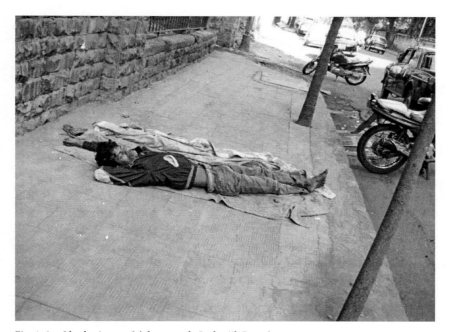

Fig. 4: Am I bothering you? (photograph: Lodewijk Brunt)

---

3   When observing sleepers and taking their pictures I always assumed they were sleeping, whatever the individual cases may be. I realise that for a real scientific approach to sleep this is hardly sufficient. There is nothing I can do about this. The suggestion by one medical sleep researcher that I should 'ring' my sleepers with actigraphs before taking their pictures is totally absurd.

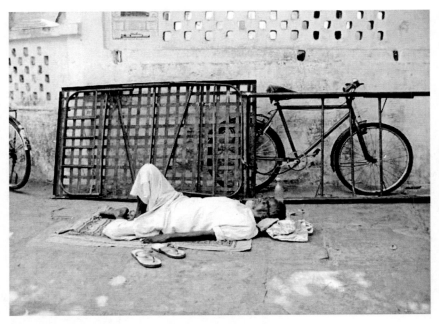

Fig. 5: Who needs the bed? (photograph: Lodewijk Brunt)

Yet in the whole of my photo collection these free spirits are only a tiny minority. Although countless millions of people spend their whole lives on the pavements of India's metropolises, many make more or less special arrangements for public sleeping. Most people have props of some sort they use for sleeping: newspapers, shawls, pillows, boxes and similar things. And, symbolically, they withdraw from public life by first taking off their shoes before they go to sleep, even if they only walk on cheap and worn-out chappals. Only once or twice have I seen sleepers wearing shoes. In India sleeping, even 'rough sleeping', is obviously connected with some sort of spiritual or perhaps religious significance – very similar to the habit of taking off one's shoes when entering homes, temples or places of ceremony. This form of 'privatisation' is often underlined by sleeping in places which are more or less separated from traffic and crowds, like small parks or pleasure grounds, benches or medium-height walls, chairs or means of transport (rickshaws, handcarts, trucks, lorries). Another way of securing some privacy is napping in groups – either groups of workers, families or collections of mothers and children. Those groups form symbolic 'islands' in the public domain of the city, which are acknowledged by passers-by. Sometimes one member of the group acts as a guard, remaining awake and looking around while the others sleep. This is especially the case in extended groups with women and children. To what extent these forms of co-sleeping have to do with (the feeling of) vulnerability is difficult to ascertain. One must not forget, however, that in terms of street crime Indian metropolises are in general much safer than cities in Europe and, especially, the United States. Of course robberies, vandalism, fighting, theft or similar forms of harassment do occur, but in no way does it have the almost epidemic character it has in other parts of the world.

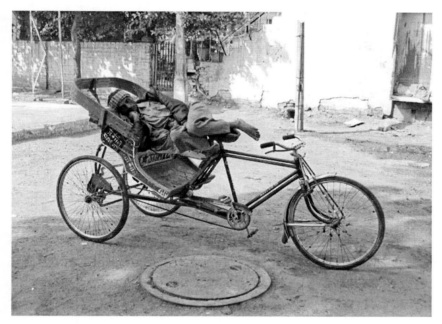

Fig. 6: Waiting for customers (photograph: Lodewijk Brunt)

Privacy is also realised by literally sleeping 'under cover'. This cover can be an arm covering the sleeper's face, but also a small towel or a blanket of any sort. On many photographs it is plain to see that people look for 'hidden spots' in the public domain. I took one picture of a man lying asleep in the middle of a parking lot, but mostly one sees people (men, but occasionally also women) lying under trees, on benches, against walls or behind objects. More often than not, sleepers have turned their backs on the crowd as well.

The fact that most people who sleep in public are poor does not make much difference for my 'theoretical' notions. It has no bearing on the overall pattern of sleep as far as I'm concerned. In my view sleeping in the streets – day or night and in every conceivable spot – is not fundamentally different from sleeping at home or even at work. In general, people move in or out of sleep easily. A very interesting point is that even in a liberal napping culture people still seem to have definite thoughts about how they should sleep and with whom. Even in the extremely crowded streets of Mumbai, Delhi or Kolkata people remove their shoes before dozing off and look for some sort of privacy, however shallow and – indeed – symbolic. In as far as India can be characterised as a napping culture – and to some degree this does not seem to be too farfetched – this does not imply that sleeping is a form of anarchy. Public sleeping in India answers to some regulations, however implicit. It does seem of importance to try and unravel these underlying norms and values. I suspect they will throw some light on the public domain in Indian cities in general, and also on the precarious balance between public and private life.

But we should not overlook that even in a standard Western sleep culture, where people sleep eight hours during the night, rules and practices are different according to the time of day. In general night time (in cities) seems to be less rigid than day time, also where sleep is concerned (Steger and Brunt 2003; Brunt 2003). People who are up and about, be it for bare necessity, professional reasons or just for fun and entertainment, seem to have liberal thoughts about when and where to sleep if the need arises. In the 1930s and 1940s, Weegee photographed a number of people sleeping on the streets of New York. In the Berinson Collection (Weegee 2007) there is a picture of at least eight men (among whom several soldiers) sleeping in an open-air eatery on the corner of Broadway and 47th Street – at 5 a.m.. In another picture two ladies and a gentleman are sleeping on the beach at Coney Island, obviously also early in the morning. There is also a wonderful picture of a small child sleeping in a telephone booth. '10 shots for 10 cents' is the title of a photo of a gentleman sleeping on a chair in front of a closed store, whereas on a similar picture a man is sleeping in front of a music store. There is a young cowboy sleeping on a bench and there is an amazing picture of six men sleeping in a car. Weegee has taken several pictures of the porch of the Wood & Selick bakery and confectionary store where single people or small groups are sleeping on a regular basis. And the most telling picture is perhaps the cellar of a building in which a couple of giraffes are being held in a cage. In front of the cage there are several mattresses lying on the floor, on which some men are sleeping. The photograph is called '*Chacun dort où il peut*' (Everybody sleeps where he can).

Conclusion

Although I'm not able to present systematic and clear-cut data, my more- or less-informed impression is that in India one finds afternoon sleeping, napping throughout the day, and sleeping just at night next to one another and perhaps sometimes overlapping. Most of my educated friends in Mumbai, for instance, all from families employed in the post-industrial sectors of Mumbai's economy, are monophasic sleepers. I think first and foremost by dictation of their work. Self-employed or employed in banks, production companies, publishers, insurance firms, newspapers, hospitals, universities. They are supposed to be present at daytime – often much longer than just from 9 till 5. Unless they are able to take naps in between their activities they are supposed to be present and at the company's service as long as they are on the company's premises. The self-employed have a business to run. The owner of a bookstore and a publishing firm I know, simply must to be present at his shop from morning till night. If there are no visitors or clients, of course, he can take naps when he feels like it. And that is what he does. Sometimes his father minds the store. Several times I came by and noticed the elderly gentleman sitting in front of the store taking a nap – within a yard or so from the deafening traffic which passes by along the narrow street.

Middle-class housewives and small children, by contrast, often have ample time to sleep during the day and that's what they do – their husbands and school-going children are away most of the day. I assume the situation to be perhaps somewhat different in the countryside regarding farmers and farm labourers. Seasonal influences might count more there than in the city, one would think. In the same vein I think there might be differences in sleeping patterns according to profession, class, caste, income, education, sex and age. In India, moreover, would climate not be of some influence as well? I wouldn't be surprised to find different sleep cultures in the mountainous regions of the north and the hot, tropical parts of the south, the great plains and the coastal areas, respectively. We have to do research; there is so much we simply don't know. As far as I'm concerned sleep research in India has still a long way to go. However, it is better to make some kind of start among the rather confusing multitude of sleeping habits, than to just continue sleeping without making any start at all.

Bibliography

AYYANGAR, KEERTHANACHARYA SREENIVASA (1991) *The Ramayana of Valmiki* (Rendered into English Prose in 2 Parts). Madras: The Little Flower.

BHAGAVAD GIITAA (2001) *Bhagavad Giitaa. Het heilig boek van de hindoes. Vertaling uit het sanskriet door Gerda Staes* (The holy book of the Hindus. Translated from sanskrit). Leuven: Davidsfonds.

BRUMMELEN, PETER VAN (2007) "'En wat liggen wij hier te doen?" De verstrekkende gevolgen van in slaap sukkelen op een bankje in het park' ('And what do we do lying down here?' The far-reaching consequences of having dozed off on a bench in the park), *Het Parool* 1 September: 12.

BRUNT, LODEWIJK (2003) 'Between Day and Night: Urban Time Schedules in Bombay and Other Cities', BRIGITTE STEGER AND LODEWIJK BRUNT (eds) *Night-Time and Sleep in Asia and the West. Exploring the Dark Side of Life.* London and New York: RoutledgeCurzon: 171–191.

CHAUDHURI, AMIT (1991) *A Strange and Sublime Address. A Novel and Nine Stories.* London: Heinemann.

CHUGHTAI, ISMAT (2006) *The Crooked Line* (Translated from the Urdu by Tahira Naqvi). New York: The Feminist Press.

DALRYMPLE, WILLIAM (1993) *City of Djinns. A Year in Delhi.* London: Flamingo.

DESHPANDE, SHASHI (2004) *Moving On.* New Delhi et al.: Penguin, Viking.

GANDHI, MOHANDAS K. (1957) *An Autobiography. The Story of My Experiments With Truth.* Boston: Beacon Press.

GUPTA, J.C. AND S.B. GUPTA (1999 eds) *Ashok Standard Illustrated Oxford Dictionary.* Sixth Revised Edition. Delhi: Ashok Prakashan.

IRVING, JOHN (1995) *A Son of the Circus.* London: Corgi Books.

KASHIKEY, RUDRA (1997) *Tales of Banaras. The Flowing Ganges. The Life and Lore of India's Sacred City on the Ganges* (Translated from Hindi by Paul R. Golding). Delhi: Book Faith India.

KOUL, SUDHA (2002) *The Tiger Ladies. A Memoir of Kashmir.* London: Review.

LAHIRI, JHUMPA (1999) *Interpreter of Maladies.* London: Flamingo.

MISHRA, PANKAJ (2004) *An End to Suffering. The Buddha and the World.* London, Basingstoke and Oxford: Picador.

MISHRA, PANKAJ (2006) *Temptations of the West. How to be Modern in India, Pakistan and Beyond.* London, Basingstoke and Oxford: Picador.

NARAYAN, R.K. (1955) *The English Teacher.* Mysore: Indian Thought Publications.

NARAYAN, R.K. (1958) *The Guide.* Chennai: Indian Thought Publications.

NARAYAN, R.K. (1993) *Salt & Sawdust. Stories and Table Talk.* Delhi et al.: Penguin Books.

NARAYAN, R.K. (1995) *The Indian Epics Retold. The Ramayana. The Mahabharata. Gods, Demons, and Others.* New Delhi et al.: Penguin Books.

NIRANJCHANA, SHAKTI (2001) *The Web of Silk and Gold.* New Delhi et al.: Penguin Books.

PATHAK, R.C. (1939 ed.) *Bhargava's Standard Illustrated Dictionary of the English Language.* Twelfth Edition. Banares: Bhargava Book Depot.

PRAWER JHABVALA, RUTH (2000) *East into Upper East. Plain Tales from New York and New Delhi.* London: Abacus.

RAKER, JOSEPH W. AND RAMA SHANKAR SHUKLA (1995a eds) *Star English-Hindi Hindi-English Dictionary.* New Delhi: Star Publications.

RAKER, JOSEPH W. AND RAMA SHANKAR SHUKLA (1995b eds) *Hippocrene Standard Dictionary English-Hindi Hindi-English.* New York: Hippocrene Books.

ROY, NILANJANA S. (2004 ed.) *A Matter of Taste.* New Delhi et al.: Penguin Books.

RUSHDIE, SALMAN (1995) *Midnight's Children.* London et al.: Vintage; originally published by Jonathan Cape, London 1981.

SCOTT, PAUL (1977) *Staying On.* London: Heinemann.

SINGH, KHUSHWANT (2002) *Truth, Love & a Little Malice.* Delhi: Penguin.

STEGER, BRIGITTE AND LODEWIJK BRUNT (2003) 'Introduction: Into the Night and the World of Sleep', BRIGITTE STEGER AND LODEWIJK BRUNT (eds) *Night-Time and Sleep in Asia and the West. Exploring the Dark Side of Life.* London and New York: RoutledgeCurzon, 1–24.

UMRIGAR, THRITY (2006) *The Space Between Us.* London: Fourth Estate.

WEEGEE (2007) *Weegee dans la collection Berinson.* Paris: Musée Maillol, Fondation Dina Vierny.

WOLPERT, STANLEY (2001) *Gandhi's Passion. The Life and Legacy of Mahatma Gandhi.* New York: Oxford University Press.

'It's Bedtime' in the World's Urban Middle Classes: Children, Families and Sleep[1]

Eyal Ben-Ari

This chapter seeks to explore the seemingly simple everyday occurrence of putting children to bed. I proceed from the following proposition: although a host of very good studies of childhood have been produced during the last two decades or so and while the scholarly literature on sleep is slowly accumulating, little work – apart from scattered studies of sleeping patterns – has been done to integrate these two bodies of knowledge. An attempt at such integration may contain a number of interesting insights into the ways in which childhood is understood and acted upon in contemporary societies and cultures. In order to situate my paper in relation to contemporary scholarship let me briefly address two questions.

Why sleep? Steger and Brunt (2003) suggest that we talk about sleep almost every day, telling our families how we have slept or wishing them a good night's sleep. Moreover, according to various time-use surveys conducted worldwide, sleep is the single activity occupying by far the largest segment of everyday life. And, in addition, the sheer amount of resources invested by families in industrialised societies in beds and bedrooms, furniture and lighting, linen or sleep clothing is staggering. But there is more to sleep than the sheer quantitative investment of time and resources in this activity. Sleep is, at once, among the most intimate, arguably one of the most personal, of activities that humans take part in and very much a socially constructed one. As Caudill and Plath (1986: 247) point out, if 'a third of our life is passed in bed, with whom this time is spent is not a trivial matter'. As they and other scholars (Gottlieb 2002; Small 1998) propose, sleeping customs seem to be consonant with major interpersonal and emotional patterns of family life in a culture. But because of its special character, sleep is more than an important manifestation

1   I would like to thank the participants in two workshops for their comments on earlier drafts of this article: one on 'Children and Sleep' was held at the University of Warwick in June 2005 and the second on 'New Directions in the Social and Cultural Study of Sleep' took place at the University of Vienna in June 2007. In addition, I would especially like to thank Brigitte Steger, Edna Lomsky-Feder, Simon Williams, Nick Crossley and Christopher Pole for their suggestions.

of emotions and social relations. Sleep is probably the ultimate phenomenon of release from pressures. People are released not only from external pressures like social ties and demands, but also from the internal pressures of our psychological forces. Sleep, in other words, allows us to retreat from everything that is 'objectively' and 'subjectively' social (Schwartz 1973: 20). Take the plethora of rules that surround the sleeping person: for example, where and when to sleep, or by whom and how one can be disturbed. In terms of the release of internal forces, sleep and the period just before sleep are relatively open to the rise of associations, thoughts, and memories whether they are pleasurable or unpleasant (Csikszentmihalyi and Graef 1975). Sleep is thus an activity or experience marked by fragility and fracturability (Ben-Ari 1996; Williams 2007).

Why children and sleep? Childhood is often considered the most vulnerable period of a person's life and arguably the stage with the greatest implications for that person's long-term cognitive, emotional and social development. Moreover, in almost all cultures of the world the birth of children is seen as a significant event for the parents in particular and for society in general and considerable resources are devoted to the socialisation of youngsters (Schwartzman 1978: 18). In regard to the focus of this article, for example, research has consistently shown that sleep is directly related to the development of memory functions and has indirect effects on cognitive development and emotional growth (Crawford 1994). Moreover, because sleep encompasses the psychological and the social, the individual and the communal, and the bodily and the cultural it would appear to be of central importance for any investigation of socialisation. In the same vein, since it lies at the intersection of meanings and emotions, sleep is also a prime site for holistically and comparatively exploring the complex experiences involved in being a human being. Yet, as Williams, Griffiths and Lowe (2007) underscore, despite the fact that sleep and sleeping are a key part of childhood and parenting, this subject has received remarkably little scholarly attention. In fact, most scholarly works that have been carried out in this regard have either been rooted in medicine with a strong focus on sleeping disorders or psychological with a great stress on concerns about why children are not getting enough sleep (Wiggs 2004).

In this chapter, I would like to take the discussion in a peculiarly 'cultural' direction. In the urban middle class of the Euro-American societies we find a particular pre-sleep bedtime 'ritual' that is (ideally) characterised by certain features. First, it usually takes place within the nuclear family and, more often than not, is part of the matri-centric model of childcare in which the mother is seen as the primary caregiver (Gottlieb 2002). Second, it is centred on the relatively private space of a separate bedroom which, if possible, is allocated to an individual child. Third, it includes a patterned set of activities: consuming an evening meal, bathing or washing, putting on special clothing, surrounding the child with special toys, telling stories and singing of lullabies, a gradual diminution of external stimuli, tucking or coddling the child in bed in a sort of 'womb', and then leaving the child alone in its room. Finally, bedtime is often seen by parents as the last chance to make this a happy, comforted and safe occasion – whatever has gone on during the day – so that children are made to feel good again. What seems to happen is that this sequence of structured and familiar processes gradually conveys the child between the states of 'wakefulness' and 'sleep' (Ben-Ari 1996).

In characterising this set of processes Small (1998) uses the notion of 'bedtime rituals', Williams (2007) echoes her by referring to 'pre- and post-sleep ritual, routines and (habituated) practices' and Kugelberg (1999: 150) suggests the idea of 'bedtime ceremonies'. The use of such imagery, however, grants the bedtime sequence of activities too strong a connotation of formality, strict procedures and explicit organisation. A better conceptualisation may be that of a 'key cultural scenario' (Ortner 1973) – alternative concepts are 'script' or 'schema' (D'Andrade 1992) – of bedtime in contemporary Western urban middle-class cultures. Key scenarios according to Ortner (1973) are valued because they formulate a culture's basic means-ends relationships in actable forms. They may be formal, usually named events, or sequences of action that are enacted and re-enacted according to unarticulated formulae in the normal course of everyday events. This conceptualisation underscores the fact that not much has to be done (minimal cues) for these actable forms to be actualised by people. In this sense, the bedtime scenario enacted by many members of current-day middle class families is something that they do 'naturally', that is habitually and unreflectingly. The bedtime scenario thus appears to be linked to certain (usually unquestioned) cultural assumptions about providing a home with security and a sense of belonging, parent-child bonding, the inculcation of certain values through storytelling and singing of songs, and a stress on health and cleanliness. Indeed, it is interesting that despite this being an era of shift work and multiple forms of families, assumptions about the nuclear family and the 'natural' and 'desired' form for putting children to sleep continue to be strong. But the key scenario of bedtime also provides a narrative structure discussing sleep and a set of criteria for appraising sleep (or its lack) and for 'correcting' it. In this sense, the scenario is used as a template for doing such things as talking, evaluating, prescribing, and medicating sleep.

In this chapter I suggest ways of examining this taken-for-granted scenario from three interrelated perspectives: an examination of how it is actually put into practice in Euro-American societies, a comparative investigation of the historical and cross-cultural differences in putting children to sleep, and an exploration of the manner and extent by which the scenario has been globalised. These perspectives may help us to integrate the questions and findings of a variety of disciplines such as sociology and psychology, anthropology and history, cultural studies and folklore, education and literature, or architecture and demography.

Bedtime in the Euro-American Middle Class

Bedtime as a social form has its own particular internal patterns and dynamics: sociologically speaking, certain rules, schedules, and spaces characterise it. To begin with, in most Euro-American societies, the bedroom is related not only sleep but also to privacy. Indeed, the link between 'bed' and 'room' connotes a separate space and a particular piece of furniture for sleep by specific individuals. This (ideal) spatial organisation is based on the Western middle class assumption of having a space for 'one's self'. Indeed, a child's bedroom is the one 'official' place of some privacy and a place where there can be at least some expression of individual taste (Mitchell and Reid-Walsh 2002: 113). What is more, in many middle class groups in such societies, contemporary coupledom is predicated on sleeping together as a symbol and expression of their relationship: 'to sleep with one's lover or partner, moreover, denotes a level of trust, intimacy and mutual vulnerability over and above the purely physical, carnal and sexual act' (Williams 2007). In contrast Japanese couples frequently sleep with their children between them,

> ... because it is considered 'natural' and 'good' to do so. From a very early age an American child is expected to become aware of the special relationship between his parents by the existence to the master bedroom with its double bed, by watching their intimate interaction, and by knowing that after a certain hour in the evening he is sent to his own room so that the

© Frank & Timme   Verlag für wissenschaftliche Literatur

adults can spend time together. Japanese children experience nothing of
the sort, and mother and her young child are often thought inseparable
twenty-four hours a day. (Tanaka 1984: 231)

Sleep and the activities related to it are thus closely related to a host of deeply
held cultural beliefs. One such idea is related to how many middle class Euro-
American parents train – or try to train – their infants to take a small and
predictable number of long naps and finally to sleep in the night for progres-
sively longer intervals without waking (Gottlieb 2002). This pattern is linked to
certain assumptions and practices related to modernity and its central values
of predictability and reliability (Melbin 1987). And the emphasis on predictability and control of the sleeping process is, in turn, connected to the ability of
parents to join the workforce and 'integrate' children into their careers as soon
as possible. Patterns of childcare, as Ennew (2002: 340) reminds us, are part of
the ways in which industrial societies use clock time and chronological age to
structure social relationships (Ennew 2002: 340).

Another conviction, propagated in many parts of the Euro-American
world, is the promotion of independence which is thought to be achieved
through the provision of a separate bedroom for a child and the pattern by
which he or she is left alone to sleep during the night (Abel et al. 2001; Gottlieb
2002). Indeed, Thevenin (1993) suggests that the general acceptance of this
generic 'male' perspective as the 'correct' one lies underneath the stress on
inculcating individual autonomy through sleep related activities. Another
relevant conviction is centred on gender. Consider how, within the bedroom,
clothing, decorations and colour schemes are marketed separately for boys and
girls (Mitchell and Reid-Walsh 2002: 128). We can thus propose that infants
routinely grow and mature within aesthetic practices divided according to
gender. Another idea now closely related to the bedtime scenario is that of
'quality time' which has been adopted in many societies as a central cultural
icon. Sleep and bedtime are now often thought to be those 'special' times that
busy middle class parents devote to children.

On a more general level, Schwartz (1973: 27) suggests that the component
of a person's identity known as 'residence' is based on a definite spatial location, normally the sleeping location. Thus

... a person 'lives' where he sleeps; even more a person belongs where he
sleeps; sleep establishes where the person is in social as well as spatial

terms; it situates him in accordance with membership rather than mere
presence and thereby generates an identity for him. (emphasis in original)

Because belonging encompasses aspects of both cognition and emotion, people are (in a sense) where and whom they sleep with. As American psychologist John Selby points out, 'one of the findings in insomnia research in the last couple of decades has been that insomnia almost always is associated with a disruption of one's sense of communal security and belonging' (Selby 1999: 7).

This point, of course, underscores the fact that bedtime is not only an individual matter for it is seen as one primary form through which parents effect the inculcation of the warmth, comfortableness, and commitment and involvement of the family. Consider the various senses involved in actualising the bedtime scenario: hearing, sight, smell, and touch. During the twilight period just before falling asleep children undergo an experience of sinking, of being submerged in a special world which in the ideal Euro-American model is that of the nuclear family. Moreover, it is within the general ambience of naptime that they exhibit – without fear of sanction or control – many private behaviours performed before sleep such as finger sucking, singing, playing with their fingers, or touching different parts of their bodies. This is no mean point, because despite the fragility and fracturability of sleep, for the majority of children, the atmosphere during sleep-time is relaxed enough for resting. Theoretically, an analysis of bedtime thus allows us to explore what Abu-Lughod and Lutz (1990: 12) term 'embodied experiences' of children, experiences that involve the whole person, including the body. In this manner we may understand how what is learnt at home becomes compelling to the children, or – to borrow from Strauss (1992: 1) – how cultural messages – such as the importance of the mother-child bond or the independence of the individual – 'get under the children's skins'. In less abstract terms, my argument is that bedtime allows us to understand how cognitive meanings become emotionally charged.

Yet sleep, and this issue is very conspicuous in regard to children, is also related to intergenerational power differentials and struggles between parents and children (Williams 2005: 79–80). Against this background we may begin to ask about children as independent actors who participate in their own socialisation: they are not merely passive beings who need to 'learn' culture. Thus for example, following Mitchell and Reid-Walsh (2002: 123) consider how although age is related to agency via the bedroom:

... clearly the infant or toddler has virtually no say over space, while the older child is gaining some autonomy over his or her own space. Thus the rooms of infants and young children ... are not really private spaces the way the bedrooms of older children, adolescents, or adults might be; rather they are more likely to be reflections of adult taste – or 'repositories' of what parents want for their children. Given that the baby's room is often decorated even before the birth of the baby, it can even become part of the home tour. (Mitchell and Reid-Walsh 2002: 123)

In a converse manner, bedrooms can be 'decoded' both for the choices made by children and parents and for the commercial intrusion into this purportedly 'private' space (Mitchell and Reid-Walsh 2002: 122).

In this regard, it may be argued that many of the social sciences have tended to project onto all children a rather peculiar view: as pre-social or pre-cultural individuals which require the actions of adults to turn them into 'full' members of society (Toren 1996). By beginning from an assumption about the 'necessity' of engaging in developmentally appropriate behaviours in order to learn to function in society, many previous studies conceptualise children as being somehow 'incomplete'. To follow MacKay's (1974) formulation, youngsters are variously immature, irrational, incompetent, asocial, or acultural all depending on whether you are a teacher, sociologist, anthropologist, or psychologist. According to this view children are seen as 'needing' to be brought up, to be completed according to adult notions of what it means to be complete. The consequence of this situation is that there is little research which seriously takes into account the role of children as active and independent agents who participate in socialisation. In contrast to these views, the child now is understood to be an agent, actively engaged in constituting the ideas and practices that will inform its adult life (James 1993; Toren 1996: 94). Interestingly, it is in and around sleep time that children's ability to bargain, struggle and resist is often very discernable, and a few exploratory studies (Williams, Griffiths and Lowe 2007) have underscored the kinds of negotiations that, depending on age, go on within families in and around bedtime.

Many psychological studies have documented the differing propensities of people to sleep at differing times and in various circumstances: for example, 'morning' or 'evening' persons or children who nap only twenty minutes a day (Lavie 1991). These differing patterns raise the question of how the family as a unit is synchronised to individual rhythms in ways that satisfy individual needs and habits. Berger and Luckmann (1967: 203) propose that socialisation does not simply involve the intrinsic problems of learning, because 'the child resists the imposition of the temporal structure of society on the natural temporality of his organism. He resists eating and sleeping by the clock rather than by the biologically given demands of the organism'. The importance of this point is not only that some children resist the patterns imposed on them by parents as part of an intergenerational struggle, but that from the latter's point of view, these children become 'problems'. Indeed, ethnographers (Kugelberg 1999: 151) report that many parents encounter children refusing to end the day by going to sleep.

Parents' responses to these problems reveal both the 'organisational' bases of administering bedtime, and how there may be a conflict between the need to react sensitively to children's needs and the need to adjust them to the family's routines (Kugelberg 1999: 150). Experts, for their part, often label the resistance of children to sleeping alone or waking up and seeking companionship as 'problems' that deviate from the belief that children should be alone in their beds at night (Thevenin 1993). Even more widely, parents may be judged in terms of whether their children are getting 'enough' sleep whatever that means (Williams, Griffiths and Lowe 2007).

The bedtime ritual is also the focus of intense activity on the part of a host of social experts such as psychologists, social psychologists, educational specialists, or medical doctors (the mythological Dr Spock). It is these experts who propagate various prescriptions and products related to the key scenario through a variety of journals and newspapers, radio and television shows, or meetings and consultations (Clarke-Stewart 1978; Kugelberg 1999: 150). A few examples are such books as *Nighttime Parenting: How to Get you Baby and Child to Sleep* (Sears 1999), *Good Night, Sleep Tight* (West with Kenen 2006), or *The No-Cry Sleep Solution* (Pantley 2002), or such web sites as *ParentCenter.Com* or *ParentsPlace.Com*. Such experts are often mobilised to analyse, write and disseminate ideas about how sleep deprivation can lead to lower cognitive achievement, attention deficiency, hyperactivity and violence. It is they who recommend that the more a child participates in creating the content of the routine, the more she or he will feel in control and responsible for her/his bedtime (and in this way hint at the importance of understanding the child as agent). They often recommend a low light for children anxious about total darkness or to prevent a child who wakes from feeling disoriented. And, in this manner, of course they have a central role in the process by which certain Euro-American cultural assumptions are reproduced through the bedtime ritual.

The very activity of diverse experts attests, I would argue, not only to the contested nature of bedtime but also the empirical variation in actual sleeping patterns. Thus, although the solitary sleeping of the young is a 'Western' invention, according to an assortment of surveys cited by Thevenin (1987) and Ball and her colleagues (1999) even today significant minorities of American and British parents routinely allow their children to sleep with them. Moreover, patterns of co-sleeping may be initiated (that is instigated by parents) or reactive (to children's demands or difficulties) (Ball et al. 1999). Other variations include moves between familial spaces (for instance, when guests visit), children migrating between the houses of divorced parents, or sleepovers. Yet despite the fragmentation of family forms and how children's sleeping arrangements are indexical of these shifting locations (Williams, Griffiths and Lowe 2007), what is common to all of these variations is that they are almost always measured against the key scenario. Thus as Ball and colleagues (1999: 149) note, parents who had co-slept with their children 'sometimes harboured sever anger or resentment towards third parties (health professionals, relatives, strangers) who voiced the opinion that parents and infants should not co-sleep, feeling passionately that co-sleeping with their infant was "natural"'.

In addition, variations on the bedtime scenario are related to the competitions and tensions related to social status. Thus for example, families may use distinctive aspects of the scenario to 'keep up with the Joneses, Kims, or Tanakas' so that they express their membership in a certain group or community. But such aspects may also be used as a way to 'keep the Cohens, Kawalskis or Chatterjees down' by explicitly or subtly emphasising anything from expensive bedroom furniture, through books, and on to the application of the latest expert advice.

Comparative Perspectives: Other Times and Other Cultures

Yet the key scenario of bedtime should not be taken as some kind of historical constant. Childhoods vary between historical periods and cultures and the ways in which we understand and organise the lives of young people vary accordingly. My suggestion is that the key scenario we have been depicting (and the practices related to it) is closely related to the emergence of the concept of childhood in Western societies. The French historian Phillippe Ariès (1962) was the first to show that modern Western childhood is unique in the way it 'quarantines' children from the world of adults. But it was only when new ideas about privacy began to appear in the nineteenth century that housing changes began to reflect these transformations and private sleeping rooms began to emerge. Accordingly, prior to the nineteenth century, co-sleeping in families and even among strangers was common; as was individual daytime sleep (Shahar 1992: 102). Since then, however, most people in Western societies have been trained to sleep alone from early childhood. In the late nineteenth century, as Stearns and his associates (1996: 345) show, sleep was absent from discussions about childhood and manuals that were mass produced for parents did not include sections about sleep. It was only later, during the 1920s, that manuals began to devote space to bedtime and that children began to be placed in individual bedrooms (Stearns et al. 1996: 357).

Given this historical diversity, we can ask how the key scenario competes with other models in other societies or other social strata within Euro-America. In Schwartzman's (1978: 9) terms every 'culture develops its own view of children's nature, and with it a related set of beliefs about how best to "culture" this "nature"'. In this respect, it would seem that the major cultural difference dividing societies is the practice of co-sleeping. In almost all cultures around the world, the norm is for babies to sleep with an adult, while older children sleep with siblings or parents (Crawford 1994; Small 1995; Whiting and Child 1953). Thus in most Asian cultures such as India, China or Indonesia private sleeping rooms are the exception rather than the rule (Steger and Brunt 2003: 12). In Japan, too, co-sleeping with family members until a relatively late age has always been very common, regardless of the number of rooms available in the house (Caudill and Plath 1986). According to this pattern, a child sleeps with its mother until the next child is born, and then she or he relocates to sleep with the father or one of the grandparents. It is not unusual for this pattern to continue until the child reaches the age of ten (Caudill and Plath 1986: 257; Befu 1971: 154–155). Indeed, research that has been carried out since the 1960s attests to the continuity of this pattern (Ben-Ari 1996).

Moreover, not only do Japanese children and parents often sleep in the same room, they often sleep on a futon. These mattresses are stored during the day, and spread out in the middle of the room with their edges almost touching during the night. In this way a parent can rather easily reach out to calm or comfort a child, and a youngster, in turn, can readily roll over and join the

© Frank & Timme   Verlag für wissenschaftliche Literatur

parent on her futon. The contrast between futon and bed as suitable places for sleep is instructive. A bed, following Caudill and Plath (1986: 267), is a separate container, an immobile receptacle. Beds usually have clear boundaries which differentiate between fixed identities. In addition, beds are usually placed at a distance from each other and for children are situated in a room separated from adults. Finally, beds are usually heavy and not amenable to easy movement. In these circumstances, caretaking often involves an effort on the part of parents who must get up and out of bed (usually moving to another room) in order to attend their children.

Even in Euro-American countries one can find the opposition between the idea of the crib to the movable cradle and the idea of individualism at bottom of the former piece of sleeping fixture (Mitchell and Reid-Walsh 2002: 124). Stearns and his associates (1996: 358) show that the separation of infants from adults for sleeping was made possible through the invention of the crib which,

> ... fenced in a young child in for sleep. They were relatively immobile, which made placement in a separate room seem both logical and essential: unlike cradles, cribs could not be moved about depending on where the parent was ... Finally, for an older infant, cribs provided safeguards from falling and wandering around ... A significant change in children's furniture ... altered the age gradations of sleeping arrangements and above all prepared the experience of sleeping alone. (Stearns et al. 1996)

Interestingly, along with the ideas of safety and individualism attached to the crib a recent addition is that notion of providing stimulation for the child and hence the development of hanging mobiles with even the bumper pads on the sides of cribs including pictures and figures (Mitchell and Reid-Walsh 2002: 125).

These differences are related, in turn, to what cultures define as proper developmental goals for children. As we saw, in most of the urban middle class cultures of the West the notion of sleeping in one's 'proper' place is related to the inculcation of independence in children (Bellah et al. 1985: 56, 57; Gottlieb 2002; Kugelberg 1999; Norman 1991: 97). Babies are often moved quite early to their own room (maybe even at the earliest possible occasion) so that they will become independent, and so that the parents may be able to enjoy some 'free' time of their own (Hendry 1986a: 21) and in order to create privacy and time for themselves (Kugelberg 1999: 150; Morelli et al. 1992). In Japan, to take one example, the emphasis is by contrast on the promotion of increasing dependence of the child on others, and primarily on the mother. In short, the stress in Japan is on cultivating mutual dependence and not independence in the sense that middle class Americans use the term (see also Tanaka 1984: 232, 233). Thus, Japanese mothers also want to promote independence but many of them believed that when they make their children feel secure by sleeping together, they will then be able to go out into the world with more self-assurance. Along these lines, sleeping in proximity to parents or on the same futon allows the creation of what the Japanese positively value as a sense of secure intimacy. According to this view, co-sleeping contributes to the fostering of dependence by reducing children's anxieties and anticipating their needs and desires. Similarly, Morelli and her co-authors (1992) point out that a Mayan mother would be shocked at the American habit of placing babies in a separate room as an indicator of them shirking their parental responsibilities of creating closeness to their children.

Globalisation: Dissemination, Power and the Key Scenario

But the question of other cultures is not 'just' comparative. Societies and the patterns of behaviour found in them are not isolated islands. Rather, there is a constant and nowadays intensified flow of ideas between them. Indeed, the idea of the child as a unique person with individual needs and abilities that parents and teachers must meet has been generalised and accepted around the globe during the twentieth century (Kugelberg 1999: 132). In some cases the dissemination of this idea has been undertaken voluntarily through emulation. In others, as Ennew (2002: 349) forcefully explains, it has been a matter of strong pressure:

> [T]hrough the work of international welfare organisations ideas of childhood are exported to the South ... Governments in countries where the children live in extended families, encouraged by foreign funding, promote the notion that correct parenting takes place only in a family with two parents, two children, and one pay packet. (Ennew 2002: 349)

To place a concrete face on this insight, one cannot understand contemporary patterns of child-care – and sleeping customs – in the Pacific region without taking into account the processes of colonisation and the variety of local patterns they created (Abel et al. 2001).

Studies of the globalisation of 'childhood', however, have tended to focus almost exclusively either on universal rights or on formal structures and organisations established to deal with children (Boli-Bennet and Meyer 1978). In this respect, it has been formal education, linked to ideologies of human rights and social progress, that has been most highly scripted with vast impact on educational expansion around the world (Meyer 2000: 234). But what about the informal aspects of education, socialisation and learning? If, to put this point by way of example, as Small (1998) and Ball and her colleagues (1999: 145) argue on the basis of data from Britain and the United States, infant sleep patterns are one of the last traditions to change under pressure from the adopted country of immigrants, then bedtime would seem to provide a very strong case for examining issues of globalisation.

Although the Euro-American pattern of putting babies to sleep may stand out as the exception among human cultures (Small 1998), we can ask about the extent and patterns by which this key cultural scenario has been disseminated to the urban middle classes of other societies such as Malaysia, Japan, Mexico or China. Lerner, Rapaport and Lomsky-Feder (2007) suggest the idea of a 'migrating script': when migrants take a script with them when moving to a new society and use it to interpret what they experience and to locate themselves in the receiving society. Our idea is of a migrating script that moves between societies to be borrowed and adapted by locals from elsewhere. Consequently, we may ask about how the 'ritualisation' of the sleep experience through lullabies, stories, special clothing, bathing and toys 'migrate' to other societies? A point made by Kugelberg (1999: 131) following Harkness, Super and Keefer (1992) is that in learning to be parents, individuals integrate their own recalled experiences of their parents with cultural models from public and informal sources and new experiences from daily life with children. In today's world, it seems that many of these parental 'ethno-models' – the interpretive schemes that parents use to understand their children's needs and development – derive from models developed in Euro-American countries.

Yet this is far from being a smooth process. The very move of the bedtime script between societies turns it into something that is not invoked automatically and thus exposes certain cultural assumptions. For example, while reading bedtime stories are an increasing part of the pattern of putting children to sleep and are often seen as an educational tool in the middle class of many non-Western societies, they are often based on traditions of oral storytelling that frequently went on during the night. In a related manner, Abel and her colleagues (2001) report that among different groups of New Zealanders, one often finds negotiated arrangements between Pacific and Maori patterns and Western ones.

The adoption and adaptation of the sleep scenario is also related to locating oneself globally. The dramatic expansion of formal schooling has tied concrete persons into globalised models of modernity by linking concrete practices to ideal images of progressive individuals (Meyer 2000: 242). But we may well conjecture that the adoption of the bedtime scenario may be seen as an act of modelling oneself on some purported ideal of Euro-American middle class-ness. In this manner, we can detect a subtle production and reproduction of a global hierarchy between different 'civilised' societies. In other words, by adopting the Euro-American model of putting children to sleep – among other practices – individuals may be signalling their global mobility into a lifestyle marked by values and practices seen as 'superior'. As Meyer (2000: 238) wryly notes, individuals 'in the modern system, consult a myriad of external rules systems (lawyers, therapists, accountants and the like) in propping up their individuality. One achieves strong status as a rational actor by becoming much like everyone else' (Meyer 2000: 238).

But interestingly, as some groups outside Euro-America have adopted the bedtime scenario, within the metropolitan West, it has actually become much more contested than in the past (cf. Ramos 2002; Wright 1997). Whether out of a harking or nostalgia for the 'past' or New Age emphases on the intimacy of the 'family bed' (cf. Ball et al. 1999), co-sleeping is seen as one remedy for the ills of an alienating modernity. Against this background it seems that the questions of 'who sleeps by whom?' (Caudill and Plath 1986) and 'where does one sleep?' continue to be important ones for individuals around the world. Accordingly, to 'go global' implies not only placing our analysis at the macro level of global processes, but no less importantly to 'go personal' to the micro level of individual consciousness and reasoning.

References

ABEL, SALLY, JULIE PARK, DAVID TIPENE-LEACH, SILATEKI FINAU AND MICHELE LENAN (2001) 'Infant Care Practices in New Zealand: A Cross-Cultural Qualitative Study', *Social Science and Medicine* 53(9): 1135–1148.

ABU-LUGHOD, LEILA AND CATHERINE LUTZ (1990) 'Introduction: Emotion, Discourse and the Politics of Everyday Life', CATHERINE. A. LUTZ AND LEILA ABU-LUGHOD (eds) *Language and the Politics of Emotion.* Cambridge: Cambridge University Press, 1–23.

ARIÈS, PHILLIPPE (1962) *Centuries of Childhood.* New York: Vintage Books.

BALL, HELEN L., ELAINE HOOKER AND PETER J. KELLY (1999) 'Where Will the Baby Sleep? Attitudes and Practices of New and Experienced Parents Regarding Co-sleeping and their Newborn Infants', *American Anthropologist* 101(1): 143–151.

BEFU HARUMI (1971) *Japan: An Anthropological Introduction.* San Francisco: Chandler.

BELLAH, ROBERT, RICHARD MARSDEN, WILLIAM M. SULLIVAN, ANNE SWIDLER AND STEVEN M. TIPTON (1985) *Habits of the Heart: Individualism and Commitment in American Life.* New York: Harper and Row.

BEN-ARI, EYAL (1996) 'From Mothering to Othering: Culture, Organization and Nap Time in a Japanese Preschool', *Ethos* 24(1): 136–164.

BERGER, PETER L. AND THOMAS LUCKMANN (1967) *The Social Construction of Reality.* Harmondsworth: Penguin.

BOLI-BENNET, JOHN AND JOHN W. MEYER (1978) 'The Ideology of Childhood and the State: Rules Distinguishing Children in National Constitutions', *American Sociological Review* 43: 797–812.

CAUDILL, WILLIAM AND DAVID W. PLATH (1986) 'Who Sleeps by Whom? Parent-Child Involvement in Urban Japanese Families', TAKIE S. LEBRA AND WILLIAM P. LEBRA (eds) *Japanese Culture and Behavior: Selected Readings.* 2nd edition. Honolulu: University of Hawai'i Press, 247–279.

CLARKE-STEWART, ALISON (1978) 'Popular Primers for Parents', *American Psychologist* 33: 359–369.

CRAWFORD, C. JOANNE (1994) 'Parenting Practices in the Basque Country: Implications for Infant and Childhood Location for Personality Development', *Ethos* 22(1): 42–82.

CSIKSZENTMIHALYI, MIHALY AND RONALD GRAEF (1975) 'Socialization into Sleep: Exploratory Findings', *Merrill-Palmer Quarterly* 21(1): 3–18.

D'ANDRADE ROY G. (1992) 'Schemas and Motivation', ROY G. D'ANDRADE AND CLAUDIA STRAUSS (eds) *Human Motives and Cultural Models.* Cambridge: Cambridge University Press, 23–44.

ENNEW, JUDITH (2002) 'Future Generations and Global Standards: Children's Right's at the Start of the Millennium', JEREMY MACCLANCY (ed.) *Exotic No More: Anthropology on the Front Lines.* Chicago: Chicago University Press, 338–350.

GOTTLIEB, ALMA (2002) 'New Developments in the Anthropology of Childhood', American Anthropological Association.
http://www.aaanet.org/press/an/0210Childcare.htm.

HARKNESS, SARAH, CHARLES M. SUPER AND CONSTANCE H. KEEFER (1992) 'Learning to Be an American Parent: How Cultural Models Gain Directive Force', ROY D'ANDRADE AND CLAUDIA STRAUSS (eds) Human Motives and Cultural Models. Cambridge: Cambridge University Press, 163–178.

HENDRY, JOY (1986) Becoming Japanese: The World of the Pre-School Child. Manchester: Manchester University Press.

JAMES, ALISON (1993) Childhood Identities. Edinburgh: Edinburgh University Press.

KUGELBERG, CLARISSA (1999) Perceiving Motherhood and Fatherhood: Swedish Working Parents with Young Children. Uppsala: Uppsala Studies in Cultural Anthropology 26.

LAVIE, PERETZ (1991) 'The 24-Hour Sleep Propensity Function (SPF): Practical and Theoretical Implications', TIMOTHY H. MONK (ed.) Sleep, Sleepiness and Performance. Chichester: J. Wiley, 65–93.

LERNER, JULIA, TAMAR RAPOPORT AND EDNA LOMSKY-FEDER (2007) 'The "Ethnic Script" in Action: The Re-Grounding of Russian-Jewish Immigrants in Israel', Ethos 35(2): 186–195.

MACKAY, ROBERT W. (1974) 'Conceptions of Childhood and Models of Socialization', R. TURNER (ed.) Ethnomethodology. London: Penguin: 180–193.

MELBIN, MURRAY (1987) Night as Frontier: Colonizing the World After Dark. New York: The Free Press.

MEYER, JOHN W. (2000) 'Globalization: Sources and Effects on National States and Societies', International Sociology 15(2): 233–248.

MITCHELL, CLAUDIA AND JACQUELINE REID-WALSH (2002) Researching Children's Popular Culture: The Cultural Spaces of Childhood. London: Routledge.

MORELLI, GILDA A., BARBARA ROGOFF, DAVID OPPENHEIM AND DEBRA GOLDSMITH (1992) 'Cultural Variation in Infants' Sleeping Arrangements: Questions of Independence', Developmental Psychology 28(4), 604–613.

NORMAN, KARIN (1991) A Sound Family Makes a Sound State: Ideology and Upbringing in a German Village. Stockholm: Stockholm Studies in Social Anthropology.

ORTNER, SHERRY (1973) 'Key Symbols', American Anthropologist 75: 1338–1346.

PANTLEY, ELIZABETH (2002) The No-Cry Sleep Solution: Gentle Ways to Help Your Baby Sleep through the Night. New York: McGraw-Hill.

RAMOS, KATHLEEN DYER (2002) 'The Complexity of Parent-Child Cosleeping: Researching Cultural Beliefs', Mothering 114. http://www.mothering.com/9-0-0/htlm/9-4-0/ramos.shtmsl.

SCHWARTZ, BARRY (1973) 'Notes on the Sociology of Sleep', ARNOLD BIRENBAUM AND EDWARD SANGRIN (eds) People in Places: The Sociology of the Familiar. London: Nelson: 18–34.

SCHWARTZMAN, HELEN (1978) Transformations: The Anthropology of Children's Play. New York: Plenum.

SEARS, WILLIAM (1999) Nighttime Parenting: How to Get you Baby and Child to Sleep. Boston: Little Brown.

SELBY, JOHN (1999) *Secrets of a Good Night's Sleep: Natural, Pleasurable Techniques Designed to Help Cure Insomnia.* New York: Universe.

SHAHAR, SHULAMIT (1992) *Childhood in the Middle Ages.* London: Routledge.

SMALL, MEREDITH (1998) *Our Babies Ourselves: How Biology and Culture Shape the Way We Parent.* New York: Anchor Books.

STEARNS, PETER N., PERRIN ROWLAND AND LORI GIARNELLA (1996) 'Children's Sleep: Sketching Historical Change', *Journal of Social History* 30(2): 345–366.

STEGER, BRIGITTE AND LODEWIJK BRUNT (2003) 'Introduction: Into the Night and the World of Sleep', BRIGITTE STEGER AND LODEWIJK BRUNT (eds) *Night-time and Sleep in Asia and the West.* London: RoutledgeCurzon, 1–23.

STRAUSS, CLAUDIA (1992) 'Models and Motives', ROY G. D'ANDRADE AND CLAUDIA STRAUSS (eds) *Human Motives and Cultural Models.* Cambridge: Cambridge University Press: 1–20.

TANAKA MASAKO (1984) 'Maternal Authority in the Japanese Family', GEORGE A. DEVOS AND TAKIE SOFUE (eds) *Religion and the Family in East Asia.* Berkeley: University of California Press, 227–236.

THEVENIN, TINE (1987) *The Family Bed: An Age-Old Concept in Childrearing.* Aldershot: Avery.

THEVENIN, TINE (1993) *Mothering and Fathering: The Gender Differences in Childrearing.* New York: Putnam Books.

TOREN, CHRISTINA (1996) 'Childhood', ALAN BARNARD AND JONATHAN SPENCER (eds) *Encyclopedia of Social and Cultural Anthropology.* London: Routledge, 92–94.

WEST, KIM AND JOANNE KENEN (2006) *Good Night, Sleep Tight: The Sleep Lady's Gentle Guide to Helping Your Child Go to Sleep, Stay Asleep, and Wake Up Happy.* New York: CDS Books.

WHITING, JOHN W. M. AND IRVIN L. CHILD (1953) *Child Training and Personality: A Cross-Cultural Study.* New Haven: Yale University Press.

WIGGS, LUCY (2004) *Children and Sleep.* Oxford: University of Oxford, Department of Psychiatry.

WILLIAMS, SIMON J. (2005) *Sleep and Society: Sociological Ventures into the (UN)known.* London: Routledge.

WILLIAMS, SIMON J. (2007) 'Dangerous/Vulnerable Bodies? The Trials and Tribulations of Sleep', CHRIS SHILLING (ed.) *Embodying Sociology: Retrospect, Progress and Prospects.* Oxford: Blackwell, chapter 10.

WILLIAMS, SIMON, FRANCES GRIFFITHS AND PAMELA LOWE (2007) 'Embodying and Embdedding Children's Sleep: Some Sociological Comments and Observations', *Sociological Research Online* 12 (5), (1360–7804).

WRIGHT, ROBERT (1997) 'Go Ahead – Sleep with Your Kids', Slate. http://slate.msn.com/default.aspx?id=2020).

Sleeping as a Refuge? Embodied Vulnerability and Corporeal Security during Refugees' Sleep at the Thai-Burma Border

PIA VOGLER

Introduction[1]

Sleep plays an important role in our physical and mental well-being. Marked by the absence of waking consciousness, sleeping persons are unable to control their environment and are therefore obliged to devise means of protection before they experience a heightened state of vulnerability (Steger and Brunt 2003: 11; Steger 2004: 355; Williams 2007: 15–17). This is even more acute in socially or economically hazardous situations, such as refugee camps in unstable border zones.

This chapter examines how forced migrants from Burma employ coping mechanisms to organise and protect themselves during sleep in a Karenni[2] refugee camp[3] located in the hilly jungles approximately 30 km outside of the town of Mae Hong Son, Thailand. I conducted fieldwork during January and February 2006 as part of an exploratory ethnographic study on livelihood strategies among Karenni refugee youth. In this study, I was particularly interested in exploring the structural difficulties faced by young refugees as well as the coping strategies they deploy in overcoming potential problems. I wanted to find out what coping mechanisms young people use when they are vulner-

---

1   I wish to thank Brigitte Steger, Lodewijk Brunt and Simon Addison for their comments on previous drafts of this paper.

2   The term 'Karenni' (red Karen) is an Anglo-Burmese term that first appeared in early colonial English literature, where it referred to an ethnic group that calls itself Kayah. Together with other ethnic groups they have proclaimed independence from Burma. The population of Karenni (Kayah) State is ethnically highly diverse. Although some of the groups are related, they often differ in language, socio-economic as well as educational background, religious practices, political aspirations and experiences of displacement. Despite this diversity, exiled persons originating from Karenni state tend to refer to themselves as 'Karenni' to lay emphasis on the (imagined) political unity of their territory (Dudley 1999, 2000:4; KDRG 2006:9; Smith 1991: 145–146).

3   Currently, there are nine refugee camps along the Thai-Burma border and the total camp population is estimated to be 150,849 persons. The site of this research is Ban Mai Nai Soi in Mae Hong Son. As of June 2006 the official population of registered refugees in this camp was 19.082 persons, mainly comprised of Karenni (TBBC 2006: 3).

able, but did not want to probe too deeply into the sensitive issues of their lives. Inspired by social studies on sleep (e.g. Steger and Brunt 2003; Williams 2005) as well as by research and reports on young people in socially and economically difficult situations (Boyden and de Berry 2004; Gigengack 2006; OCHA/IRIN 2004), I assumed that a close look at refugees' 'sleep' might provide a window to individuals' vulnerability and also their agency in providing measures for basic safety in otherwise adverse environments.

The chapter begins with the theoretical and methodological considerations that guided this study, followed by a presentation of the social and material conditions of sleep within the Thai refugee camp. I then provide four examples of how embodied vulnerability is exacerbated within this setting and point to the strategies refugees devise in order to reduce these risks and vulnerabilities. In conclusion, I suggest that investigating sleep can indeed be a very useful tool for understanding the life worlds of people in hazardous circumstances. Talking and learning about sleep is not only a sensitive approach to more sinister topics, such as domestic violence, an unstable housing, etc. Examining sleep also points out the material, mental and spiritual resources people mobilise proactively in order to protect themselves.

Theoretical and Methodological Considerations

Human beings are embodied by virtue of their existence. Far from being a static concept, embodiment designates continuous engagement with one's own corporeal identity throughout the course of a life (Turner 1984: 7, 2003: 277–278). Yet, through involvement with society, our corporeal and psychic integrity are prone to experiences of economic scarcity, emotional hardship and disease. 'Embodied vulnerability' is thus an inescapable part of the human condition: 'To be vulnerable as a human being is to possess a structure of sentiments, feelings and emotions by which we can steer a passage through the uncertainties of the social world' (Turner 2003: 277).

This condition of embodied vulnerability is particularly pronounced during minimal states of consciousness, such as sleeping and dying – when our involvement with society is (temporally) suspended (Williams 2003), or at least limited.

Therefore, in order to sleep well, individuals and groups need to make arrangements that allow for a maximum of corporeal security during sleep.

Based on extensive research in Japan and other countries, anthropologist Brigitte Steger proposes, 'the question of security is a key towards a theoretical understanding of sleep as social event' (Steger 2004: 357). Safety during sleep cannot merely be explained with reference to physiology. It is also intimately related to social, cultural and spiritual aspects at a particular time and place. (Aubert and White 1959a: 54; Steger 2004: 355).

Steger identifies four elements that facilitate emotional security cross-culturally: first, the stability of the sleeping place; second, the presence of trusted persons; third, the existence of repetitious rituals; and fourth, the social acceptance of a certain sleeping behaviour (Steger 2004: 415). While all of these factors appear to shape sleep throughout the world, their particular importance may vary in different cultural contexts.

Guided by Steger's theoretical considerations on the provision of security during sleep, I attempted to explore how Karenni refugees provide for essential protection whilst asleep.

Methodology

During this exploratory research I worked with qualitative research methods, such as participant observation, informal interviews with individuals and groups of young people and the collection of ethnographic material. In this endeavour, I encountered several methodological challenges.

First, the refugee camp as major social situation for participant observation proved to be a difficult research site. In terms of general accessibility, the obtainment of a camp pass – the official entry document to the camp – issued by the Thai Ministry of the Interior would not have been possible without affiliation with a registered organisation operating within the refugee camp. For this reason, I volunteered with a local NGO. While this was a very reward-ing experience, it also caused constraints during fieldwork. For example, introducing myself to the refugee population as an NGO volunteer and gradu-ate student sometimes caused confusion among research participants. Also, my own moves during research in the camp had to be chosen carefully in accordance with my host NGO and partner organisations on which I de-pended for transport to and from the camp (for details cf. Vogler 2007).

The imposition of curfews as artificial markers of nightfall merits special attention. According to Aubert and White, the fixation of a temporal frame for nocturnal rest serves in particular those who hold powerful daytime positions and whose temporary withdrawal from their positions while sleeping exposes them to attempts to undermine their authority (Aubert and White 1959b: 9). Similarly, imposed sleep simultaneity functions as a means of social surveillance.

At the time of research, humanitarian aid-workers had to leave Thai camp-sites by 6 p.m., while refugees had to respect an internal curfew set at 9 p.m. The latter regulation – literally a *couvre-feu* – clearly aims at curbing nocturnal traffic by requiring camp residents to cover open fires and maintain silence within their homes. Although the mere setting of a curfew does not cause refugees to go to bed obediently, it arguably defines a normative time frame for collective rest. Moreover, the curfew prescribes what kinds of persons are allowed to take a night's sleep within the camp. Like this, nightfall forcibly separates the camp population from diurnal actors such as humanitarian aid workers and researchers affiliated with them. At the same time, curfews engender proximity between refugees and other actors such as Thai paramilitaries who are deployed as night watchmen with special accommodation inside the camp (cf. Vogler 2006). Bearing ethical considerations in mind, it was impossible for me to stay overnight in the camp. Had the Thai authorities found out, this would not only have shed a negative image on the NGO I worked with, but more importantly, it would have caused grave problems for my refugee hosts.

I remedied these limitations by visiting other living areas of refugees around the camp on a daily (and nightly) basis.

Second, I found myself faced with the dilemma encountered by most social researchers focusing on sleep, namely, the fact that as an unconscious activity, sleep is difficult to account for both by researchers and research participants. In most industrialised societies, sleep qualifies as a 'hidden private phenomenon' (Hislop et al. 2005: 7.1.) thus posing practical challenges to direct observations. The privacy of sleeping persons was not a major issue in the refugee camp, since it was usually unproblematic to visit sleeping spaces in and around refugees' homes. Notwithstanding this advantage, I experienced the limits of participant observation due to my own sleepiness. For example, when refugees allowed me to take a rest on their bedding during my camp visits they did so because of my obvious exhaustion. Accordingly, I always readily and thankfully accepted these offers from my side. Because these occasions always correlated with my own drowsiness, I ended up taking notes and pictures

© Frank & Timme   Verlag für wissenschaftliche Literatur

before falling into comfortable slumber. At the same time, I had to be discrete in taking notes about the bedding as the sight of a tired person examining and writing about bedding instead of sleeping in it would have caused much amusement if not confusion!

Concerning interviews, sleep turned out to be an easygoing topic with Karenni refugees. They not only seemed to enjoy recounting childhood memories of co-sleeping or jaunty episodes of putting overprotective parents to sleep with alcohol, moreover, discussions of sleep allowed them to approach sensitive issues regarding the vulnerability and protection of individuals' corporal integrity that may be difficult to obtain when asked directly. However, ethnographic conversations and interviews were limited due to language constraints. At the time of research I did not speak any of the local languages and, therefore, interacted mostly with those who spoke English. This choice immediately limited my informants to young educated refugees. Engaging a translator would have been possible, though difficult, since people in the Karenni camp speak various languages. Furthermore, the brevity of fieldwork did not allow for sufficient time to identify a trustworthy person to engage for the delicate task of translation. Since my research also involved visiting refugees who resided irregularly outside the camp in the evening and night-time hours, I considered it safer to see people alone rather than in the company of a second person.

Finally, I also collected visual sources depicting or discussing sleep. These include photographs and drawings by refugees as well as illustrations printed in books and calendars. I also found it useful to shape my understanding of Burmese sleep habits through the analytical reading of non-academic literature describing everyday customs inside Burma. Despite their semi-fictional character, these texts proved helpful in forming initial ideas on the 'social acceptance' of sleep behaviour among Burmese refugees.

The Social and Material Conditions of Sleep in the Refugee Camp

Sleeping places inside the Thai refugee camp consist mostly of unstable bamboo huts built by refugees. The physical condition of the camp area appears to be a major obstacle for the construction of stable housing: located in the deep jungle on steep hillsides, the area designated by the Thai government does not allow for generous space between individual houses. Bamboo and eucalyptus are used as general building materials and roofs consist mostly of leaves. These materials are also customarily used for houses in rural Burma as well as in Thai villages close to the camps (TBBC 2006: 70).

Although the bamboo weakens rapidly and has to be replaced every two years, refugees are not allowed to use other building materials. The houses are therefore prone to various natural hazards. The porous roofs, walls and floors cannot truly protect the inhabitants from the weather conditions in northwest Thailand, whether the oppressing heat during March and April or heavy rainfalls during the monsoon period lasting roughly from May to September. In particular during the rainy season, landslides and falling trees might completely destroy or wash away individual bamboo huts. In addition, the permeability of the huts exposes their inhabitants to malaria transmitting mosquitoes and disturbing noises.

Despite the limited options in housing design, refugee homes – and thus their sleeping spaces – differ according to the economic status and gender composition of household members. Also, for children, birth order is an important factor structuring their sleeping location.

Economically better-off families appear to have at least one room for married couples and several other rooms for children who often share space with same-gender siblings. In the absence of an adequate number of rooms, a minimum of protection is maintained by curtains, which divide the beds of siblings, relatives, and friends who are not of the same sex. Exceptions to gender separation are married couples and pre-pubescent children. Husbands and wives tend to share either a room or a corner within the bamboo huts. Babies and infants sleep with their parents and usually leave the parental bed when a neonate joins the family. Notwithstanding this general rule, several informants mentioned that they practiced parental co-sleeping until their teenage years, in particular with their mother. One young man only ceased to share the parental bed when he reached the age of fifteen (Oh Thay[4], personal communication, 13 January 2006). Michael, another refugee, recounted the emotional hardship caused by his exclusion from the parental bed at the age of nine: 'I was cryin', is cold and lonely.' (Michael, personal communication, 13 January 2006). Pitying their younger brother, Michael's older siblings started to shelter him alternatively under their blankets. Since one of the siblings was an older sister it can be assumed that co-sleeping among different genders is not problematic

....

4   All names of research participants are pseudonyms.

during childhood. By contrast, unmarried adults are expected to sleep separately. In general, the co-sleeping of adult men and women is only permissible for a married couple within their own household. A household is considered 'polluted' if any other couple shares bedding in a home that is not their own. Therefore, overnight guests usually sleep in groups of men and women with children joining the female group for sleep. It is uncommon to provide a private sleeping place for invited couples or families. Within Karenni state itself, whole villages may visit each other for major celebrations. At these occasions, the host villages provide men and women huts to shelter the people of the invited village (Reh Mi, personal communication, 29 November 2007).

Verandas also appear to be used for both nocturnal and diurnal sleep. If a household does not possess enough space, visitors are asked to spend the night on the veranda. The same holds true for families who lack space and who send their sons 'outside' to sleep with friends. Moreover, I observed sleeping or dozing men, women and children on their verandas during the early afternoon hours.

While the above descriptions concern sleeping places within individual households, many young refugees are sheltered in boarding houses and schools run by different organisations and charities. These establishments mostly house unaccompanied minors who arrive at the camps. In these boarding houses and schools male and female students sleep in separate buildings. Boys sleep in an open dormitory with beds located next to each other in a long row on the wooden floor. This pattern is not peculiar to refugee camps, but can also be found in orphanages for migrants in Mae Hong Son and in Buddhist orphanages inside Burma. In contrast to their male peers, girls are sheltered in buildings that allow for more intimacy. Usually two to three girls are allocated one room. Teachers explained these different spatial arrangements with reference to the need for privacy, which is supposedly more pronounced among girls. Yet, according to another informant, male students of this boarding school complained about their sleeping places and asked repeatedly for dormitories in the style of their female peers (Maude, personal communication, 29 November 2007).

Sleep items such as clothes and bedding often serve the immediate purpose of protecting the sleepers' corporeal integrity. Moreover, their usage may also hint at reassuring rituals that either facilitate one's falling asleep or are 'called forth by the latent fears which may be aroused by the imminence of sleep' (Aubert and White 1959a: 50).

Similar to refugees' sleeping places, there is also a variety of bedding used inside the camp. In general, NGOs provide refugees with blankets, non-impregnated bed nets and plastic sleeping mats. The common distribution rate consists of one blanket for every two refugees as well as one family-size bed net and one sleeping mat per three persons. During unusually cold winters, refugees may also receive knitted blankets. Used in conjunction, the mats and nets provide an essential protection against wind and malaria transmitting mosquitoes.

Apart from official aid material, refugees develop their own strategies to create comfortable bedding. Although pillows are not among relief items, cushions exist in almost every household. Furthermore, women, children and men support their heads with bunches of clothes and logs. These pillow alternatives should not be interpreted as a sign of poverty, since cushions are not commonly used in Burma (Thanegi 2004: 35).

Most refugees sleep on the floor by putting a thin mattress on a plastic mat and by covering themselves with distributed blankets. Depending on their economic situation, they may acquire additional items such as quilts and thicker blankets either by purchase them from shops within and outside the camp or by bartering. During the daytime the bedding is usually removed in order to provide space for other activities. According to research participants this is even the case in households with specifically allocated sleeping rooms. In the absence of drawers and other furniture, mats and blankets are folded into neat packages and stored at discreet posts in the hut.

In addition to blankets and quilts, refugees protect their bodies directly with their clothes. It is noteworthy that the practice of wearing clothing reserved for nocturnal sleep does not exist among the Burmese refugees. Instead, women and men sleep in their *longyi*[5] or other clothes worn during the day.

Sources of Vulnerability and Means of Protection

Four key elements are likely to cause distress that may prevent refugees from sleep or interrupt their slumber in an unpleasant if not perilous way, namely: the permeability of bamboo huts, the refugee community, the militarisation of

---

5   A *longyi* is a sheet of cloth, often sewn in a cylindrical shape. It is worn around the waist and runs to the feet. *Longyi* are worn by both men and women in countries like Burma, India, Bangladesh and Sri Lanka.

       © Frank & Timme   Verlag für wissenschaftliche Literatur

refugee camps as well as the belief in supernatural beings. Yet, despite the threats these elements signify for individual sleepers, they function simultaneously as protection against other hazards.

As described above, housing within the refugee camp consists of bamboo huts, which are not only characterised by the poor quality of building material but also by unavoidable neighbourly proximity. It does not take much to imagine the impact that these conditions have on sleep and nocturnal tranquillity.

First of all, informants repeatedly mentioned the sounds of human activities and animals. While morning sounds related to peoples' household chores seem to be accepted as part of the day's start, sounds during night time have rather been identified as disturbing sleep. For example, several refugees reported being woken up in the morning as soon as their neighbours began woodcutting as well as feeding pigs and chicken. Indeed, wood cutting is one of the first morning activities, since it is indispensable for the preparation of morning rice. Rather than as disturbing 'noise', the sounds of morning work should therefore be interpreted as 'background sounds' marking the transition from the dormant to the waking condition. Those responsible for these morning chores are not necessarily working in silence but usually start chatting in normal voices. There seems to be no social rule requiring 'consideration for the neighbour' during early morning hours. By contrast, other noises such as snoring, footsteps in neighbouring bamboo-huts, or the noises of roosters and frogs were described as nocturnal sleep disturbers. Furthermore, my co-worker Julian mentioned that camp residents would call security personnel if drunkards were too loud (Julian, personal communication, 21 January 2006), while a refugee woman reported a 'crazy' woman who would sit on the roof of her hut during full-moon nights singing the whole night through (Ree Meh, personal communication, 25 January 2006).

Second, refugees and foreigners who happened to spend nights with official permission in the camp complained that the permeability of the bamboo huts exposed them to harsh weather conditions during sleep. For example, a Swiss civil engineer mentioned the noises of footsteps and an unpleasant draught going through the gaps of the floor and walls when he spent a night inside the camp during his consultancy (Henri Stalder, personal communication, 19 February 2006). An Austrian NGO worker experienced similar exposure during her stay in the camp two years ago and came to the conclusion that a night in a bamboo hut is like sleeping in an 'open cardboard box' (Gabriele Schaumberger, personal communication, 4 January 2006).

Acute health-related problems may arise during the monsoon period when constant rainfall endangers those who are sleeping under leaky roofs. In an attempt to counter this hazard, refugees have developed various techniques for sealing roofs. I observed people using blue plastic sheets or blankets distributed by NGOs to cover holes in the roofs. As protection from malaria transmitting mosquitoes, bed nets used in conjunction with plastic mats are invaluable relief items and as such are regularly distributed by NGOs. Yet, notwithstanding their protective function, mosquito nets may also become fire dangers. Apart from sleeping, refugees also pursue other nocturnal activities under their bed nets such as learning and reading. In the absence of electricity they use candlelight, which is likely to burn the nets. At the same time, the permeability together with the proximity of bamboo huts may also provide social protection by virtue of neighbourly vigilance.

Domestic and gender-based violence constitute the single largest group of offences committed in refugee camps around the world (Da Costa 2006: 10). This holds true for the refugee camps alongside the Thai-Burma border. Women and children, in particular, live with the threat of various forms of sexual harassment, and other forms of violence, which more often than not are perpetrated by members of the refugee community, including of one's own household.

Social studies on the impacts of domestic violence in other settings have found that abusive relationships are likely to cause sleep problems that may persist even long after victims and perpetrators have been separated. For example, a study with women in British shelters highlights that forceful sleep deprivation is often part of domestic abuse. The disturbed sleep of women may moreover translate to the sleeping behaviour of children living in the same household (Williams 2005: 134).

The account of a Thai social worker responsible for child-centred programmes in Mae Hong Son confirms these findings. Apparently many Karenni children experience difficulties falling asleep due to quarrelling parents (Thiphawan Teethong, personal communication, 20 January 2006).

Sleeping women may also be vulnerable to assaults committed by nocturnal prowlers. For instance, anthropologist Sandra Dudley describes how during her research stay in a Karenni camp an unknown man supposedly repeatedly sneaked into all-female households – including her own – molesting young sleeping women. The first attempts to catch the prowler consisted of male youths moving into the concerned bamboo houses where – equipped with sticks and stones – they spent the night in the public areas of these households.

Yet, their protective efforts remained unsuccessful. The problem of the nocturnal intruder persisted and was even aggravated when refugees started to ascribe these machinations to supernatural beings (Dudley 2000: 274).

Notwithstanding the potential danger embodied (mostly) by male members of the refugee community, refugees also find emotional comfort through the presence of others during sleep provided that dormant bodies are decently covered and arranged properly according to gender. As mentioned above, Karenni refugees neither change into sleeping clothes nor sleep naked. They keep on wearing their clothes, but are supposed to arrange these carefully in order to cover their skin while asleep during daytime and night-time. Both genders manage to wrap their clothes tightly around their waists thus ensuring that the fabrics will not move during sleep. This holds especially true for refugee women who are expected to cover their legs down to the ankle with their clothes and an additional blanket. According to refugee Moe Nyo, female friends and relatives are expected to re-cover a dormant person should the *longyi* or blanket be misplaced. By contrast, if men – other than husbands – observe an uncovered woman, they may look away, move on or ask someone else to re-cover the dormant body. Moe Nyo, furthermore, indicated that the sight of such a 'messy' sleeper might appear ridiculous to the beholder: 'In their heart they will say something. They want to laugh' (Moe Nyo, personal communication, 12 January 2006). Among Karenni women, the wrapping and tightening of their *longyi* therefore seems to function as a primary sleeping ritual.

In contrast to the sleeping demeanour of women in visible places, the shelter of one's bamboo hut seems to allow for more relaxation. Thus, while men and boys appear to have greater freedom in choosing their sleeping place and are sometimes even sent outside to spend the night on the veranda, girls and women are encouraged to seek the privacy of the bamboo hut for a decent sleep.

Although not located in an open combat zone, the ongoing atmosphere of civil strife and political violence translates from the Burmese to the Thai side of the border and thus into the refugee camps. Also, with the exception of those already born in Thailand, refugees are likely to suffer from sleep disturbances caused by memories of individual experiences of armed conflict and internal displacement.

Research among refugee children from the Middle East in Denmark by Edith Montgomery and Anders Foldspang (2001) suggests that a violent family history in conjunction with a continuing stressful family situation may serve as a strong predictor of sleep disturbances. The authors found that while long-lasting exposure to violent environments enhances the likelihood that children will live in a constant state of arousal, sleep disturbances are mainly the result of witnessing or experiencing more specific incidents of violence (Montgomery and Foldsprang 2001: 21).

It has to be kept in mind that the above research findings apply to a specific group of refugee children and, therefore, cannot simply be generalised to other contexts of forced migration. Notwithstanding this limitation, these insights suggest that a research focus on sleep may reveal how experiences of structural and direct violence are likely to continue haunting individuals for a very long period.

In contrast to the resettled children in the above case study, everyday life of Burmese youth in Thai camps occurs in proximity to the ongoing civil strife within the Burmese jungles. This also explains the strong politicisation and militarisation of these camps. Between 1995 and 1998, for instance, refugees and Thai locals alike suffered from an estimated 152 cross-border attacks of the Burmese Army and its allies. Refugee camps constituted the main target of these assaults (including five camps that were completely burned down), since the Burmese Army suspected them to be strongholds of non-state armed groups (Lang 2002: 154–156). Partly as a result of these cross-border attacks, Thai paramilitary sentries were installed for the first time within the camps in 1997 (Bowles 1998: 12).

Yet, far from being perceived as exclusively protective, the presence of Thai security personnel may impact negatively on peace of mind during nocturnal hours and, thus, on the sleep of some refugees. Accounts of Thai soldiers aggressively treating individuals strolling around after curfew hours, on the one hand, and cases of refugee girls entertaining romantic relationships with Thai soldiers, on the other hand, are likely to stir parental fear that may prevent household elders from falling asleep. Compared with the Karenni boys, the Thai soldiers are socially well off, they wear uniforms and move around on motorbikes and thus attract the attention of quite a few girls. Since the soldiers are, however, unlikely to marry their Karenni girlfriends, parents are concerned about these relationships. For example, when I discussed the issue with a group of young refugees, it transpired that parents tend to worry if their daughters do not return between 10 p.m. and midnight (Group discussion, 17 January 2006). Because these hours are already far beyond the fixed curfew hours, the group discussion also suggests that official regulations do not necessarily hinder refugee youth in their nocturnal projects.

In contrast to the somewhat ambiguous role of Thai soldiers, the Burmese Army continues to be perceived as a serious threat by the refugee population and those working with them. During fieldwork, several people recalled in detail the last serious engagement between the Burmese Army and the Karenni Army. The armed clash took place during the 2005 dry season as the absence of rain facilitated Burmese soldiers' access to Karenni territory:

> During that time the sound of gunfire and explosions was a daily back-drop and a curfew was imposed in the camp. Every night everyone had to be home and candles out by 8 p.m. for fear of the Burmese invading the camp (they have done it before so this was not an imagined threat). There was real fear in the camp and the curfew also impacted on study and en-tertainment. At that stage our boarding master refused to take in any new students as he was finding it so difficult to control the boarder students, as they were so restless. (Maude, email-correspondence, 26 March 2006)

During a group discussion, students also spoke about this period. Recounting the fighting at the border, a male student mentioned how insecure he and his friend felt because of the sounds of shelling and gunshots. An aid worker who lived inside the camp at that time confirmed that the shelling was audible in particular during the evening and early night hours (Mary, personal communication, 21 February 2006). Many refugees had already packed their belongings and remained in a constantly alert state. They were ready to leave the camp at any moment (Group discussion, 21 February 2006).

These accounts suggest that fighting does take place during evening and night time and that this hazard may impact on refugee's sleep. At the same time, it transpired that the presence of Thai soldiers – originally meant for protection – might also be perceived by some members of the refugee community as a nocturnal threat to their peace of mind.

Parallel to Theravada Buddhism as the official state religion, animist beliefs in supernatural beings are widespread in Burma. In particular the belief in *nats* is very popular. According to anthropologist Melford Spiro (1996) '*nat*' refers to a class of supernatural beings who are more powerful than humans and who can affect them either for good or for evil (Spiro 1996: 41). Together with witches, ghosts and demons, *nats* constitute a system of supernatural beings that appear to play a salient role in the everyday life of most Burmese, including ethnic minorities (Spiro 1996: 4).

Although *nats* are believed to possess the power to affect human beings in various ways and situations (including sleep), humans are not passively subjected to the whim of ethereal creatures. Instead, people can irritate but also appease supernatural beings. Accordingly, while one remains vulnerable to the deeds of malevolent *nats*, the belief in miraculous things can also provide protection and refuge from mental distress caused by the empirical world.

Yet, while waking agents are capable of keeping supernatural machinations at bay, sleepers seem to be particularly vulnerable to ghostly visitations. For example, during fieldwork in Burma anthropologist Monique Skidmore encountered a woman who claimed that the ghost of her husband would haunt her every night (Skidmore 2004: 202). Also, the former Karenni refugee Pascal Khoo Thwe recounts in his autobiography his grandfather's ghost paying his sleeping wife and grandchildren a visit (Khoo Thwe 2002: 93–94). Years later, when the young man lived and studied in Cambridge, his troublesome past continued to manifest itself during dreams and caused him nights of fitful sleep. Similar to the resettled refugee children researched by Montgomery and Foldspang (2001), direct experiences of political persecution and violence continued to trouble Pascal long after he had left Burma, once his consciousness ceased to follow wakeful discipline and started operating according to the opaque regulations of the dormant condition. Since he was in exile, recourse to indigenous healing methods in order to soothe these spiritual torments proved to be impossible.[6] The situation was further exacerbated by the fact that he could not confide in his British colleagues due to his fear of being misunderstood:

> *Ghosts and nightmares returned to haunt my nocturnal world. Sometimes my ancestors visited me to offer their blessing, while at other times evil Nats haunted me and bullied me into giving up the struggle. The ghosts of dead friends came often to my assistance, and the goodwill of living ones was a balm of my horrors. Yet, much of the time I felt that I was under the*

....

[6] In this respect, it is noteworthy that there exist examples of extreme repercussions of spirit belief that are summarised as Sudden Unexpected Nocturnal Death Syndrome (SUNDS). Since the 1970s, SUNDS has been striking Hmong and other Southeast Asian refugees and migrants in their sleep. Medical anthropology explains these nocturnal deaths with Southeast Asians' geographical detachment from their ancestors' lands and ghosts and the resulting spiritual dilemma (Adler 1995: 1626).

spell of evil powers I could not talk about any of this to my friends. They had no conception of our 'ghost culture', of how we took for granted things that to them would have seemed quaintly superstitious or mad. (Khoo Thwe 2002: 278–279)

Sleep, therefore, constitutes a particularly vulnerable condition for those holding animist beliefs. Accordingly, keeping potentially sleep-disturbing fears and dangers at bay, requires the performance of special rituals. For example, if we return to Sandra Dudley's account of nightly intrusions into her and other women's bamboo huts, Dudley further reports that after a while most refugees were largely convinced that these incidents were caused by *nats* who had been offended by the camp community. At this point the majority of the camp population was already alert and extremely disturbed by these stories that accompanied ongoing incidents of nocturnal intrusions. Eventually, an end to the intrusions was only achieved through the intervention of a shaman (Dudley 2000: 275–276). Remarkably, this was an effective way to expel the intruder.

Emotional security, however, may also be reinforced through concentration on or complete immersion into the spiritual world itself. The Burmese intellectual Ma Thanegi, for instance, describes *nat*-storytelling as a helpful strategy when sending children to sleep (Thanegi 2004: 27–28). Striking indeed are Skidmore's accounts of Burmese citizens deploying supernatural beliefs as coping mechanisms within an environment severely characterised by structural violence. According to her study, individuals apparently manage to withdraw from distress by putting themselves intentionally into unconscious states such as sleepwalking, daydreaming and soul wandering (Skidmore 2004: 188–199).

Concluding Remarks

While sleep in general puts the body into a state of vulnerability, this is particularly pronounced in the case of refugees. In this article I outlined how Karenni refugees in Northern Thailand devise coping mechanisms in order to protect their corporeal and mental integrity during sleep. I argued that the sleep of forced migrants is, on the one hand, overshadowed by certain vulnerabilities and dangers. On the other hand, I suggested that far from being mere victims to adverse circumstances, refugees are capable of developing mechanisms and strategies in order to cope with potential sleep-disturbing elements.

Steger's (2004) theoretical framework on emotional security during sleep proved very helpful in discerning aspects of refugees' vulnerability and agency. Indeed, the findings of this study suggest that issues she identified – stability of sleeping places, presence of trusted persons, existence of repetitious rituals and social acceptance of sleeping behaviour – are also relevant for sleep within the refugee camp. Observations of refugees' sleeping places illustrate how camp inhabitants have to work continuously on the maintenance of the stability and impermeability of their bamboo huts. Refugees' comfort during sleep seems also to be enhanced by the presence of trusted persons, whether friends or relatives. The necessity of the social acceptance of a certain sleeping behaviour is illustrated by strict rules separating sleepers according to gender. Furthermore, I explained how Burmese women, in particular, are expected to avoid the demeanour of a 'messy sleeper' by adequately covering their body. There are also rituals that support individuals' smooth transition into the dormant state and back into a waking condition: spreading out one's bedding may already be an important ritual as well as the obligatory adjustment of cloths for proper sleep. Moreover, research findings thus far suggest the existence of religious rituals meant to abate the negative influence of supernatural beings upon sleepers.

This research found a frequent blurring of the distinction between elements causing 'vulnerability' and those signifying 'protection': What some may experience as nuisance (e.g. exposure to sounds due to the permeability of bamboo huts), may be perceived by others as protection from more sinister dangers (e.g. escalation of domestic violence). More research is needed on the impact of social categories such as age, gender and class on the organisation of refugees' sleep. Thus far, research on Karenni refugees' livelihoods suggests that refugee women sleep less than their male counterparts due to domestic obligations. Moreover, men tend to be less occupied due to the official Thai prohibition of paid labour and agricultural work for refugees. In particular, engagement in paid labour can have a strong impact on the organisation of refugees' sleep since this activity often causes refugees to leave campsites secretly under the veil of darkness (cf. Vogler 2006).

Methodologically, I found 'sleep' a useful window for further explorations of social settings marked by political and economic adversities as well as structural inequality and injustice. Yet, this was not always an easy process. Exploring the provision of emotional security during sleep within the Karenni refugee camp was complicated by the research context as well as by the condition of sleep itself. Official regulations as well as the particularity of sleeping

© Frank & Timme   Verlag für wissenschaftliche Literatur

situations rendered constant observations very difficult. At the same time, approaching sensitive issues through sleep-centred conversations, interviews and observations proved very fruitful. In particular, it had the advantage of being less obtrusive and probing than more direct inquiries into peoples' intimate lives and fears. Indeed, while talking about sleep, refugees recount at their own pace details about their social relations, their emotional vulnerabilities as well as protection mechanisms.

Therefore, I am convinced, that further research on sleep of 'vulnerable populations' can provide important insights into individuals' vulnerability and also into their agency in providing measures for emotional security in otherwise adverse environments.

References

ADLER, SHELLEY R. (1995) 'Refugee Stress and Folk Belief: Hmong Sudden Deaths', *Social Science and Medicine* 40(12): 1623–1629.

AUBERT, VILHELM AND HARRISON WHITE (1959a) 'Sleep: A Sociological Interpretation I', *Acta Sociologica* 4(2): 46–54.

AUBERT, VILHELM AND HARRISON WHITE (1959b) 'Sleep: A Sociological Interpretation II', *Acta Sociologica* 4(3): 1–16.

BOWLES, EDITH (1998) 'From Village to Camp: Refugee Camp Life in Transition at the Thailand-Burma Border', *Forced Migration Review* 2 (August): 11–14.

BOYDEN, JO AND JOANNA DE BERRY (2004 eds) *Children and Youth on the Frontline: Ethnography, Armed Conflict and Displacement*. Oxford: Berghahn Books.

DA COSTA, ROSA (2006) *The Administration of Justice in Refugee Camps. A Study of Practice*. Geneva: UNHCR (= Legal and Protection Policy Research Series).

DUDLEY, SANDRA (1999) 'Traditional Culture and Refugee Welfare in North-west Thailand', *Forced Migration Review* 6: 5–8.

DUDLEY, SANDRA (2000) *Displacement and Identity: Karenni Refugees in Thailand*. Unpublished D.Phil. thesis. University of Oxford.

GIGENGACK, ROY (2006) *Young, Damned and Banda. The World of Young Street People in Mexico City, 1990–1997*. Amsterdam: Universiteit van Amsterdam.

HISLOP, JENNY ET AL. (2005) 'Narratives of the Night: the Use of Audio Diaries in Researching Sleep', *Sociological Research Online* 10 (4). http://www.socresonline.org.uk/10/4/hislop.html (accessed 4 March 2008).

KDRG (= KARENNI DEVELOPMENT RESEARCH GROUP) (2006) *Damned by Burma's Generals. The Karenni Experience with Hydropower Development*. Chiang Mai: KDRG.

KHOO THWE, PASCAL (2002) *From the Land of Green Ghosts. A Burmese Odyssey*. London: Harper Perennial.

LANG, HAZEL J. (2002) *Fear and Sanctuary. Burmese Refugees in Thailand*. Ithaca: Cornell Southeast Asia Program (= Studies on Southeast Asia 32).

MONTGOMERY, EDITH AND ANDERS FOLDSPANG (2001) 'Traumatic Experience and Sleep Disturbance in Refugee Children from the Middle East', *European Journal of Public Health* 11(1): 18–22.

OCHA/IRIN (= UNITED NATIONS OFFICE FOR THE COORDINATION OF HUMANITARIAN AFFAIRS/INTEGRATED REGIONAL INFORMATION NETWORKS) (2004) *'When the Sun Sets, we Start to Worry …'. An Account of Life in Northern Uganda*. Nairobi: OCHA Regional Support Office for Central and East Africa.

SKIDMORE, MONIQUE (2004) *Karaoke Fascism. Burma and the Politics of Fear*. Philadelphia: University of Pennsylvania Press.

SMITH, MARTIN (1991) *Burma: Insurgency and the Politics of Ethnicity*. London and New York: Zed Books.

SPIRO, MELFORD E. (1996) *Burmese Supernaturalism*. New Brunswick and London: Transaction Publishers.

STEGER, BRIGITTE (2004) *(Keine) Zeit zum Schlafen? Kulturhistorische und sozialanthropologische Erkundungen japanischer Schlafgewohnheiten*. Münster: LIT.

STEGER, BRIGITTE AND LODEWIJK BRUNT (2003) 'Into the Night and the World of Sleep', BRIGITTE STEGER AND LODEWIJK BRUNT (eds) *Night-time and Sleep in Asia and the West. Exploring the Dark Side of Life*. London: RoutledgeCurzon, 1–23.

TBBC = THAILAND BURMA BORDER CONSORTIUM (2006) *Programme Report: January to June 2006*. http://www.tbbc.org/resources/2006-6-Mth-Rpt-Jan-Jun.pdf (consulted November 2006).

THANEGI, MA (2004) *The Native Tourist. A Holiday Pilgrimage in Myanmar*. Bangkok: Silkworm Books.

TURNER, BRYAN S. (1984) *Body and Society. Explorations in Social Theory*. Oxford: Basil Blackwell.

TURNER, BRYAN S. (2003) 'Biology, Vulnerability and Politics', SIMON J. WILLIAMS ET AL. (eds) *Debating Biology: Sociological Reflections on Health, Medicine, and Society*. London and New York: Routledge, 271–282.

VOGLER, PIA (2006) 'In the Absence of the Humanitarian Gaze: Refugee Camps After Dark', *New Issues in Refugee Research* 137. Geneva: UNHCR.

VOGLER, PIA (2007) 'Into the Jungle of Bureaucracy: Negotiating Access to Camps at the Thai-Burma Border', *Refugee Survey Quarterly* 26(3): 51–60.

WILLIAMS, SIMON J. (2003) 'Liminal' Bodies? Sleep, Death and Dying', SIMON J. WILLIAMS ET AL. (eds) *Debating Biology: Sociological Reflections on Health, Medicine, and Society*. London and New York: Routledge, 169–181.

WILLIAMS, SIMON J. (2005) *Sleep and Society. Sociological Ventures into the (Un)known*. London and New York: Routledge.

WILLIAMS, SIMON J. (2007) 'Vulnerable/Dangerous Bodies? The Trials and Tribulations of Sleep', CHRIS SHILLING (ed.) *Embodying Sociology: Retrospect, Progress and Prospects*. Oxford: Blackwell, chapter 10.

'Early to Rise': Making the Japanese Healthy, Wealthy, Wise, Virtuous, and Beautiful

BRIGITTE STEGER

Every morning, some 240,000 commuters stream out of the train stations in the bustling Tokyo office district of Marunouchi and start their exhausting workday, already full of stress from their long commute in the crowded train. An '*asa expo*' (morning expo) has been held biannually since autumn 2006 (www.asaexpo.net) to help these people start their day with enjoyable activities. A number of workshops on topics such as yoga or coffee brewing, along with concerts and lectures are meant to help business people feel relaxed and prepared for the day's high demands. One of the initiators, Furuta Hima, believes that this 'may be the beginning of a whole change of lifestyle and [...] work-life balance' (Hani 2007).

This 'morning expo' seems to be part of what 'mental journalist'[1] and industry consultant Ōmika Naoko has called a 'recent trend in adult early rising' (Ōmika 2006). However, the morning expo group is not the first promoting early rising and morning activities. The demand to rise early can be found in some of the earliest written Japanese sources and has been repeated throughout history, similar to other parts of the world, such as China, India and Europe.

In fact, most of the historical texts that advocate early rising in Japan were influenced by Confucianism and Buddhism. In her study of notions of sleep in early Chinese texts, Antje Richter (2001: 111–124) points out that 'late to bed and early to rise' was usually sufficient as a description of proper Confucian conduct. In Buddhism, the desire to sleep (*suimin-yoku*) had to be suppressed in much the same way as the desire to eat/drink or to have sex, be it that sleep was less prominent in the discussion (cf. Kaibara 1995: 26, 28, 38–39, 48; Mochizuki 1967: 1385–1386). Early rising has been promoted in school textbooks for the elite samurai class as well as the ones for commoners, such as the *Dōjikyō* (widely in use from the early sixteenth to the late nineteenth century).

---

1   The term seems to have been coined by Ōmika herself in English; apparently her connotation is that she writes on mental well-being.

The lines children had to learn to read and write by heart read like follows: 'Mornings, get up early and wash your hands, evenings go to bed late and wash your feet' (Kurokawa 1977: 11).

Early rising is one of the most prominent topics in the literature dealing directly or indirectly with sleep. By contrast, bedtime has attracted much less attention. In Japan, moreover, from the early twentieth century onwards, 'early-rising associations' (*hayaoki-kai*) have been active throughout the country. In the 1990s, in bookstores I found shelves full of advice books promoting early rising, and currently one can find entire websites and campaigns devoted to the issue.

Taking into consideration that during sleep one is 'dead to the world', it is obvious that sleep is a threat to rational social order (see also Cox in this volume). Simultaneously, however, humans need to sleep as preparation for the performance of their duties. Thus, regulating and limiting sleeping time, especially in the morning, when sleep can be both recuperation and indulgence, and exercising a certain degree of control over the transition from the private sleep to the performance of social duties, is an important way of integrating bodies into social life. This chapter will expound on these theoretical considerations by paying attention to the ways in which nationally organised early-rising associations in the first half of the twentieth century, and current early-bird activities in Japan try to control both the rising times and the transition phase of many people. Furthermore, by analysing arguments and movements that promote early rising both historically and for contemporary Japan, I will investigate the changes and continuities of what early-rising promoters consider to be the performance of social duties.

My sources are mainly house codes, textbooks and regulations as well as medical publications for pre-modern times, and publications by early-rising associations, how-to books and websites on early rising as well as interviews and visual material for modern and contemporary periods. I have conducted two years of field work on sleep from 1994–1996 and have subsequently returned to Japan regularly, most recently in December 2007, to generate new data and continue to delve into the issues that the analysis of the interviews and written sources revealed as central to sleep research.

'Early to Bed, Early to Rise – Makes a Man Healthy, Wealthy and Wise'

In pre-industrial societies, daylight saving was quite understandably important. However, the notion that people went to bed at sunset and rose at dawn is
incorrect. The court life of the nobility described in the literature of the Heian
period (794–1185) was primarily night life. Even the less affluent were up
during hours of darkness, especially in winter when the days were short. If the
harvest had to be collected because of a weather change, farmers stayed out in
the fields to get the job done without question, even when the stars and the
moon were the only sources of light. Moreover, with the promulgation of the
Keian no ofuregaki (Ordinances of the Keian era; 1649), peasants had to
perform night work (*yonabe*). *Yonabe* generally implied performing routine
tasks at home that did not require much light, such as weaving, lacing, and
mending and was to be performed in addition to field work. Nevertheless,
wasting precious fuel was generally frowned upon, in particular in those social
groups where frugality played an important role, such as among peasants and
merchants. The most central themes emphasised in all house codices of
mercantile families were diligence, frugality, obedience towards the government, and preservation of the reputation of their houses (Ramseyer 1979: 210).
Those who rise early are able to use the whole day for work and also prove
their integrity, which promotes the reputation of the house or family. Apart
from that, early rising prevents wasting money. For salespeople, waking early
meant that they would then go to bed earlier and not spend money on oil or in
the pleasure quarters. At the same time, they were sure to get their work done
properly. One of the oldest of these house codices, from the merchant Shimai
Sōshitsu from Hakata written in 1610, *Shimai monjo*, states:

> Get up early in the morning, and do the same in the evening [i.e., go to
> bed early]; one shouldn't waste oil for unnecessary tasks. One shouldn't
> stay awake without having an important reason. (Itō 1972: 54)

The existence of such directives informs us not only about the social desirabil-
ity of early rising, but also that even in pre-modern times, people would not
necessarily have found such directives 'natural' and easy to obey. Especially
young people found it difficult to get up early.

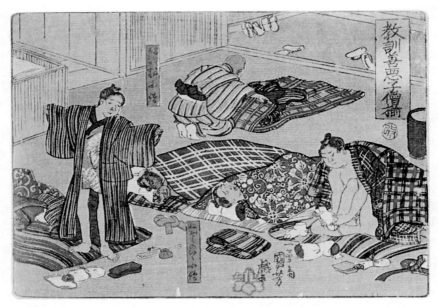

Fig. 1: Caricaturist Utagawa Kuniyoshi in his satirical series on good and naughty apprentices (1857) depicts two well-behaved apprentices who are sleeping in on their (rare) holiday, while three ill-mannered apprentices – usually getting up late – are exceptionally keen to get ready to visit their family early in the morning. Courtesy, Sepp Linhart.

What is early? The sources reveal that there is no consensus on this issue. Rising times range from 'when it was still dark' to sometime around sunrise. In general, rising times for members of the lower classes were earlier. They typically had to start their working day at dawn, often around the 'sixth hour', which was defined as the time when daylight made it possible to see the deep, strong lines in the balm of one's hand, but the small lines were still invisible. Rising schedules and night-time sleep length thus varied depending on the season and the eyesight of the person who tolled the bell (for a detailed discussion cf. Steger 2004: 286–294). In any case, the exact hour of rising is and was secondary. Most of the directives do not even give a specific hour. Early means that one should rise earlier than usual, earlier than other people and first of all, not indulge in leisurely 'morning sleep'.

Compared to Benjamin Franklin's 'makes a man wealthy', the Japanese promise, '*hayaoki wa sanmon no toku*' (early rising yields three *mon*; a very small currency unit, no longer in circulation), is modest. It does not promise sudden wealth, but instead makes it clear that one must work hard in order to increase wealth little by little. *Toku* is written with the Chinese characters for 'merit', but is a homophone of 'virtue', thus emphasising the moral aspect of early rising and increasing wealth through hard work.

Rising early, working long hours diligently and not neglecting one's duties were thus demanded in pre-modern times, but it was only after the introduction of the equinoctial time system with hours of equal length in 1873 that work time could be measured and paid by the hour (cf. Nishimoto 1997), and the money gained by early rising could be precisely calculated. As cultural historian Kuriyama Shigehisa (2002: 222) points out, the newly introduced idea that 'time is money' implies an accumulation of time. Making proper use of odd minutes here and there would add up to a veritable sum of time.

In 1925, Yamamoto Takinosuke, one of the leading figures in the early-rising movement and author of the book *Hayaoki* (Early rising), explains:

> *Early rising creates time. It extends the day's horizon. People who get up one hour earlier will have a space of one more hour per day. In one month this hour amounts to 30 hours, in one year to 365 hours. If we assume that eight hours in a day are allocated to work, and we rise one hour earlier, we gain three and a half days per month, and in one year we gain 45 days. (Yamamoto 1925: 1–2)*

The idea of saving bits and pieces of odd sleeping time in order to create new time is also common in contemporary advice books on early rising and sleep reduction. One author even speaks of seventy full days a year that one can gain from a five-hour reduction in daily sleep (Fujimoto 1995: 4–5).

The simple equation is 'less time for sleep equals more time to be productive'. These writers reject as pure nonsense the notion that people need eight hours of sleep and feel that reducing sleep is basically a matter of knowledge, will and effort. They deny that sleep deprivation can endanger health and concentration. On the contrary, by rising early one accumulates even more energy, an argument to which I shall refer below.

Some authors (e.g. Kawamura 1995: 62; Saisho 1994: 132) explain that waking earlier than everyone else enables one to open one's shop earlier and, thus, have more clients than one's competitors, but they are hardly convincing. Most jobs are performed inside the house, and artificial light is readily available.

Empirically, the time-use surveys of the NHK[2] reveal that both times to get up and times to go to bed have become postponed during the second half of the twentieth century, and they are considerably later in urban than in rural areas. Nevertheless, the energy saving argument of earlier times is gradually coming back into the discussion, but people express ecological concerns rather than economic ones. '[I]f you go to bed a bit earlier to get up early the next morning you can contribute to reducing energy consumption at night. We are not saying that morning life should be promoted for environmental reasons, but as a result we can contribute ecologically as well. And that's nice, isn't it?' concludes Furuta in his explanations of the aims of the 'morning expo' (Hani 2007).

Early rising is connected to an increase in wealth in other respects as well. However, the meaning of wealth has changed. A 'wealthy way of using the morning', which is the title of the work by the chairman of an ethics association, Kawamura Shigekuni (1995), includes making use of the morning hours for studying and learning. The title of another work, from the vice-president of an early-rising association, Kurosawa Masatsugu, suggests that 'early risers obtain qualifications in a relaxed manner'. Hereby, the author argues, one climbs one step up the ladder in the business world and social status. In addition, obtaining more qualifications opens up a new world in which other highly qualified people live, thus leading to friendships. Communication between these new friends will be highly intellectual and will stimulate further attempts to obtain even more qualifications (Kurosawa 1994: 116–117). Early rising thus enriches life intellectually, socially and emotionally. More recently, the early-bird phenomenon in Japan has begun to influence industry, reports the Taiwanese *CommonWealth Magazine* (Wu and Chang 2008), there are now 'dawn language classes' on offer so that 'office workers can learn when their minds are fresh and head straight to work afterwards.' Kurosawa (1994: 30) explains: 'The efficiency of one hour in the morning can be compared to two in the evening. There is no other time that is more ideal for studying than the early morning'. Leaving the question of efficiency aside, the authors seem to imply by promoting studying in the early morning that one should spend the most work-efficient time for one's own advancement and dream fulfilment rather than for the company. However, before people are able to fulfil their dreams, they need to know them. A range of recent books thus promotes the 'morning

---

2   The research division of the Japanese Public Broadcasting Corporation NHK has conducted large-scale time-use surveys (*NHK kokumin seikatsu jikan chōsa*) in 1941 (published in 2000) and one every five years since 1965, usually published the following year.

diary' (*asa nikki*), which includes getting up early and writing down dreams to enhance their 'dream quotient' and thus enable success (Satō 2005).

Leisure and Play in the Morning – Changing Values

Compared with earlier sources, the how-to books and campaigns for early rising no longer promote getting out of bed early for the benefit of the family, house, company or community. Arguments today emphasise the merits for the individual. Contemporary early-bird promoters even suggest filling the morning with leisure activities. A typical line of reasoning of a group of young business people and professional runs as follows:

> For everyone, a day has 24 hours and a year 365 days. How much of this time can you [the reader] really enjoy and do whatever you like? The answer to this question may shock you because you are always in a hurry and have no time to enjoy life and fulfil your dreams. The only time of the day that is not yet so full of stress is the morning. Therefore, you should consider this time carefully and use it properly. (*Gendai jōhō kōgaku kenkyūkai 1994: 3–6, abbreviated*)

Until some twenty years ago such an argument for early rising would have been unthinkable. No single older source promotes spending time and money on leisure activities in the morning. On the contrary; in 1925, for instance, Yamamoto emphasised, 'if you use [the additional time in the morning] for meaningless play, it is of no use. Even if one gets up very early but does nothing but smoke […] one would only waste tobacco and oil expenses, and should rather stay in bed' (Yamamoto 1925: 3–4). Starting the day with play was considered as a sure way to ruin one's wealth, family and reputation.

Why has there been a shift in value towards leisure? And why do business people promote getting up early so that people have time to play rather than sleeping an hour more and arriving well rested at work? The shift in values was gradually induced in the 1970s by the Japanese government's so-called 'leisure development policy'. The policy was mainly meant to support the leisure industry and was backed by the theory that in advanced post-industrial societies, the gross national product GNP was dominated by the service and leisure industries, and people would have more free time. For this reason, time and money spent on leisure began to be seen as an indicator of wealth (Linhart 1988: 274–275). In modern Japanese history, competing with the advanced nations has always been an important issue. Thus the leisure development policy killed at least three birds with one stone. First, it supported the economy by raising inland consumption and made Japan thus internationally competitive and less dependent on trade relations. Second, it showed the world that Japanese people could enjoy themselves and were thus socially advanced. And third, it satisfied the demands of people who wanted to enjoy the fruits of their hard labour.

Although the theory that post-industrial societies are more leisurely has since proved inaccurate, it nonetheless has had a great impact on the significance that people give to wealth. People are discouraged from simply lying around dozing and watching TV in their free time. Instead, they are meant to reduce nocturnal sleep, spend their time actively and discover new hobbies (cf. Steger 2004: 181–223). Leisure and enjoyment on a regular basis which had been regarded as a vice, unless confined to certain social groups, times and/or spaces, has now become almost a social duty, albeit not on the expense of neglecting other (and more important) social duties such as work and family. A socially responsible and attractive person is well rounded and knows how to enjoy him or herself.

According to the early-rising group, when one gets up an hour or so earlier, the day can begin with something pleasurable. Importantly, leisure is no longer 'left-over time' after work, when one is weary, as the Japanese term for leisure (*yoka*) suggests. It is newly created free time. By utilising this time, one goes to work in a cheerful mood (Gendai jōhō kōgaku kenkyūkai 1994: 130–135). Thus, although the emphasis in the argument is on pleasure, it is clear that the ultimate goal is to set the mood for a more engaging performance of one's duties.

Controlling Emotions

Whereas hitherto arguments deal with the questions of 'creating' time and how to spend this time, and thus point to changes and continuities in individual, social, and economic values, they do not sufficiently explain why getting up earlier rather than working, studying or playing at night would be the best way to pursue these activities. I suggest, that the morals conveyed by rising 'earlier than usual', as the website of the morning expo puts it, and regulating transition phases are central to our discussion.

The elaborations of one interviewee, Mr. Nagamatsu, a 48-year-old Tokyo ward official, on getting up during the holidays or a weekend trip are particularly revealing. He noted that in Japanese-style hotels (*ryokan*), the breakfast hours (before 8 a.m.) and check out (10 a.m.) are early, but even guests who do not want breakfast and those staying several days still get up early.

> *It might be strange, but if a Japanese does not get up early, she or he is called* darashi ga nai. *[...]* Darashi ga nai *means that this person is believed not to lead a proper life. Therefore, even if one stays awake until late, one has to get up early. If a couple slept into the day during their honeymoon, people in the* ryokan *would think, 'ah, last night they were at it for quite a while'. That is why they try to behave properly [and get up early], even when they are tired. On a company trip it is the same. Personally, I do not say so, but the older colleagues do. In the evening everybody consumes a lot of alcohol, but you must arrive early, they teach us. You must not be defeated by alcohol. Especially for working people, it is a matter of shame to be called* darashi ga nai, *isn't it? Therefore, it is a matter of honour to pretend to get up in the morning in a perfectly correct way. [...] If you appear at work unshaven, without a tie or with unkempt hair, you are also considered* darashi ga nai.

> *[B.S.:] Is this just a question of shame or does this have definite negative consequences related to the prospects of promotion or the like?*

> *It depends on each individual case whether one is able to make progress or not. But a* darashi ga nai-*person cannot be entrusted with a desirable, difficult assignment. If you ask me, I do not disagree. [...] It means that this person is not reliable. It means that they cannot put their emotions in order; order is not the right word [...] cannot control their emotions. In the end it means that the person is too weak to suppress emotions. (Interview, 19 December 1994)*

Nagamatsu's story is a good example showing that even those who stay awake until late at night have to get up early. Although the Japanese language is gender-neutral, in this case it is obvious that Nagamatsu refers mainly to his male colleagues or more generally to *shakaijin* (responsible full members of society/job holders). It is 'his' responsibility to make sure that 'he' gets sufficient sleep and is prepared for the following day. At another point in the interview, Nagamatsu makes clear that for this reason he usually goes to sleep early. Although there is considerable pressure to be social and have a drink with others at night, *shakaijin* must still maintain sufficient control over their behaviour to ensure their ability to rise early the next morning and get to work as usual. The reputation of being a 'real man' increases with the amount of alcohol consumed, but only if this does not impair the 'real man' the following morning. These are tough demands; and there is a whole industry profiting from them. About 150 different kinds of energy and vitamin drinks are available to help people recover from hangovers and sleep deprivation and carry on through the day, with roughly 1,260 million bottles sold annually. Even though women also consume energy drinks, advertisements usually address men only; and they reproduce the image of 'male power [that] may more generally be strength not only of body but also of mind' (Roberson 2005: 368, 376–378).

The consequences that Nagamatsu describes of not getting up early and thus being considered *darashi ga nai* are far-reaching. The person is not considered an honourable member of society and cannot be entrusted with a difficult assignment or responsible position. Nagamatsu himself is 'weak' in the morning and, therefore, is tolerant of late sleepers. Nevertheless, he agrees with the notion that a person incapable of controlling his or her 'emotions' is necessarily unreliable. The crucial point of early rising is thus to suppress or control one's 'emotions' or physical desires, and to be morally fortified.

Organised Early Rising

Nagamatsu's explanations express notions that were spread throughout Japan by 'early-rising associations' (*hayaoki-kai*). According to Yamamoto (1925: 125–126), the first such group was the Tōmonkai (East Gate association) or officially, the 'Young people's health raising association', founded in 1897 in the village of Hirosaki in Aomori Prefecture. Its members, all teenagers, gathered every morning before daybreak in front of the East Gate to do some physical exercises. Before the callisthenics, they sang war and other songs in a loud voice.[3] Loud singing goes back to the habit of early morning reading classes in

---

3   A similar ceremony is described in the *Nihon shoki* (720). Office hours and morning ceremony were set at the palace in Ogōri, in present-day Osaka, which was inaugurated in 647.

pre-modern schools for commoners, where pupils had to read out at the top of their lungs. The groups Yamamoto (1925: 125–194) describes were usually initiated by heads of villages and hamlets, who could draw on the *wakamono-gumi* (Edo-period young men's associations on the village level). Their explicit aim was to provide additional education for young men after they had graduated from the compulsory primary school to help them cope successfully with modern economic circumstances. Although some of these groups met in the evening, Yamamoto describes many that met at sunrise before the start of their work day.

Building on such local traditions and initiatives, after the Russo-Japanese war (1904/05) in November 1905, several senior members of the Home Ministry and Ministry of Education founded *hōtokusha* (Maeda 1999: 257, 263). *Hōtokusha* or *hōtokukai* refers to Ninomiya Sontoku, also known as Ninomiya Kinjirō (1787–1856). As an orphan at the age of sixteen, he was the breadwinner in the family, but also went to school and studied hard to ultimately become a successful agricultural expert and landowner. He even served in the Tokugawa shogunate. Using a variety of technical and socioeconomic innovations as well as ideological slogans, he taught the rural population to achieve greater yields from their crops. He also supported well-known virtues, such as honesty, diligence, thriftiness, and co-operation within the rural population. Through the creation of reciprocity-based credit unions (*hōtoku*), he made new technology affordable for agricultural workers (Havens 1983: 7–8). Sontoku remains well known today as he was a role model of virtue in school books of the 1930s. A statue of him as a schoolboy carrying a pile of wood and reading while walking was erected in front of every primary school and his face adorned the new one-yen note in 1946.

Hōtokusha soon spread throughout the rural regions. The movement promoted 'moral, economy, autonomy and education' (Maeda 1999: 258–59) of the rural communities. Japan won the war against Russia, but with 55,000 dead and 144,000 injured virtually no village was left untouched. People questioned not only the conscription policy (formerly only samurai were allowed to have weapons) and financial burdens imposed by the war, but also other policies of

---

As a rule, persons holding official rank shall draw up in lines to the left and right outside the south gate at the hour of the tiger [i.e. 3-5 a.m.]; they shall wait there for the sunrise, go to the court and bow twice. Then they shall enter the attendance hall. Those who come late will not be permitted to enter and take up their attendance. When the bell tolls at the hour of the horse [11 a.m.-1 p.m.] they may retire. The official in charge of striking the bell shall wear a red apron. The bell-stand shall be set up in the Middle court (Ujitani 1993: 181).

the new national government (Kokuni 2007: 1–2). *Hōtokusha* was the first local level, large-scale organisation successfully used by the government to ensure 'social cohesiveness and harmony' in the countryside and support for industrialisation, nationalism and war efforts (Pyle 1973: 61).

The mouthpiece for *hōtokusha* was a monthly journal called *Shimin*, which was meant to educate young people and households. *Hōtokusha* also promoted its goals via postcards. One of these cards,[4] most likely a New Year's card, deals with early rising. The card shows two pictures with a number of word games. In a circle are three *mochi* (sticky rice cakes as *shintō* sacrifices; eaten on New Year's day), *mochi* is a homophone of 'having'. *Sue* means in the end, but is a pun on the (rich) leafs of the tree. This picture describes the goals and benefits of *hōtokusha*. The larger picture is of a deeply rooted, early-rising tree, dense with leaves and fruit.

Hōtoku mi takara mochi *ichimei shiawase (kingōjō) no* *kagami mochi*	The three treasure mochi of *hōtoku* in other words: the *kagami mochi* of happiness (literally: hard work, coopera- tion and generosity)
Shōjiki na kokoro o *mochite kimochi yoku* *kasegi hatarake(ba)*	To have a sincere heart and, work hard with a good feeling
sue wa kanemochi	The end result is to 'have money'
setai motsu *fūfu* *kokoro o awasemochi* *shimatsu yoku seba* *sue wa iemochi* *kane mochite ie o tamochite* *yo no tame ni tsuki wa*	If a couple who owns a household deals with things properly together If one does it well right from the start, the end result is 'to have a family'. To have money, to keep a family, to exhaust/beat yourself for the good of others.
mitsu no takaramochi nari	This means to have the three treasure *mochi*

----

4   Details about these postcards are unknown; Sepp Linhart found the card at a Viennese flea
    market. I would like to thank him for letting me use the card. I owe gratitude to Akashi Eiichirō,
    Noriko Brandl and Richard Bowring for their help in deciphering the text.

© Frank & Timme   Verlag für wissenschaftliche Literatur

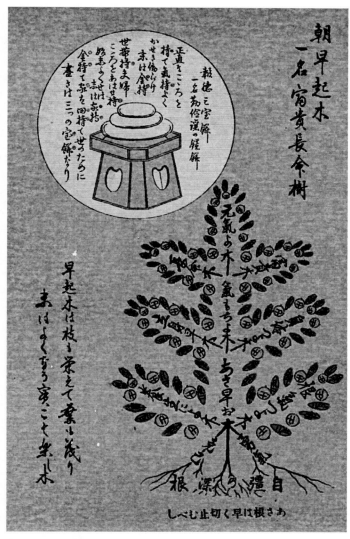

Fig. 2: The *hayaoki* (early-rising tree) by the *hōtokukai*. Courtesy, Sepp Linhart.

According to this poem, *hōtokusha*'s most important principle is working with an honest heart. Goals are material, such as the purchase of property for the rural population, but a no less important virtue is a harmonious family life. A house (*ie*) means more than just a building and refers also to a family, which carries with it a certain social status and is the administrative foundation of the modern state. Notably, the postcard does not hide the fact that *hōtokusha*'s path is very strenuous and long. But, it maintains, the toils of hard work do not bring a mere superficial, easily accessible happiness. Instead, they lead to permanent prosperity and harmonious human relationships: the basis for a stable prosperity.

The text at the roots of the tree explains: Foregoing morning sleep means cutting the tree's weak roots. This enables a deeply rooted, strong self. Early rising is the basis upon which all further virtues are built. According to this picture, the result of self-denial and courage is a healthy, sound person. Such people have all of the requirements for social and economic success, but also for being happy and virtuous.

Hōtokusha had sub-groups for young people (*seinen*) and women (*fujin*), which would both eventually become independent, national organisations (they still exist today). In 1910, Tazawa Yoshiharu (1885–1944), the later Minister of Home Affairs, officially founded the *seinendan* (young men's association); later, girl's groups were also set up. Tazawa was inspired by the activities of the already quoted Yamamoto who as a school teacher in Hiroshima had tried to persuade the Ministry of Education to promote the education of disadvantaged rural youth. One of the aims of *seinendan* was to prepare the youth to build up the nation, both economically and *in spirito* (Tani 1984: 249–252). When the Meiji Emperor died in 1912, *seinendan* from all over Japan were invited to Tokyo to build the Meiji shrine and to collect one yen from each member. This collaboration for building one of the most important national symbols promoted the rural youth's identification with the nation state. They came from all over Japan with different dialects and cultural backgrounds to share uncommon 'Japanese' food, sleeping, working and other activities as well as a common goal. This camp experience was again inspired by Yamamoto, and in later years, camps played a central role in *seinendan* activities, esp. from the early 1930s (Seinenkan 1989: 243). Also in 1912, Tazawa set up the All-Japan Seinendan Federation. The official *seinendan* history written in 1942 does not put much emphasis on early rising; but in passing it often mentions the early-rising associations or early morning callisthenics of the youth groups (e.g. Seinenkan 1989: 244, 334). According to Yamamoto's (1925: 189) descriptions, for many early-rising groups, outdoor gymnastics (in some cases called *kokumin taisō* or national gymnastics) was a central activity.

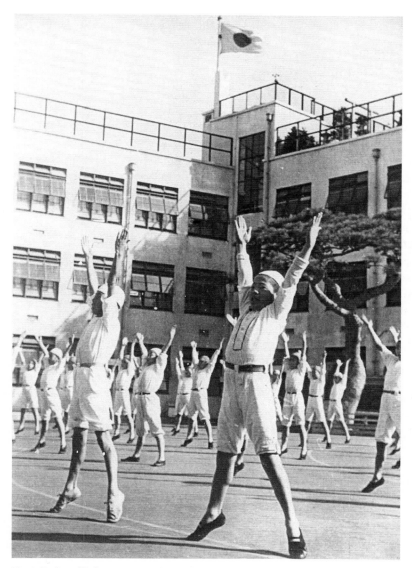

Fig. 3: Radio callisthenics, 1930s. Courtesy, Japanese Studies section of the Department of East Asian Studies, University of Vienna; photographer unkown.

In 1928, the newly established national broadcast corporation NHK introduced radio callisthenics (*rajio taisō*); the idea of broadcasting gymnastic programmes via the new means of radio came from an American insurance company (Yamashita 1999: 93), but NHK could build up on the many groups in the villages who were already accustomed to getting up early and meeting outside for physical exercise. Until today, radio callisthenics are broadcast throughout the year at 6.30 a.m.; it is especially popular among elderly people, but over the summer holidays the exercises were and are targeted at primary school children. Even if they are still very sleepy, children have to get up early in the morning, gather in the neighbourhood, do the exercises, get a stamp and go home again. For company employees, there are programmes at 8.40 a.m. (as well as at noon and in the afternoon), which enables them to exercise before they start work.

Seinendan had (and has) both socialist and nationalist elements. It gave young people in the villages an opportunity to study and advance socially. Yamamoto is said to have been inspired by the Movement for Freedom and Democracy. However, with the Ministries of Education and Home Affairs as its leaders, *seinendan* increasingly became a very strong tool to mobilise young people both in war efforts and – after the war – economic reconstruction.[5] One other widespread rural organisation was the (*Teikoku*) *zaigō gunjinkai*. These groups, literally 'local (Imperial) military groups', were intended for men after they became too old for *seinendan*. More than 11,000 such groups existed in 1910. Rather than fighting in war, they were in charge of youth group leadership, disaster relief aid, and preparation of patriotic ceremonies and other communal services (Pyle 1973: 63). Members of *gunjinkai* also had to get up early on cold winter mornings at 4 or 5 a.m., sometimes dressed with one shirt only, to do physical exercises (Yamamoto 1925: 138–142).

The managing director of *gunjinkai*, Lieutenant General Tanaka of the Imperial Army, emphasised the importance of sleep for young people. However, he argued, that since it takes a lot of courage and a self-denying spirit to get up early, especially in the cold winter, rising early will help build a firm and determined spirit. Moreover, as experience shows, early rising also leads to less

....

5   According to Kakeya Shōji, Vice-director of the research unit at the Seinenkan, the head office of *seinendan* (personal communication, 17 December 2007), some Japanese researchers argue that the Hitlerjugend was built on the *seinendan* model. Although this seems farfetched, as Germany had its own tradition of youth organisations, there is ample evidence that German representatives visited Japan and were inspired by this very successful organisation. While the Hitlerjugend was abolished after 1945, *seinendan* still exists today, but has lost its attractiveness in recent years.

socialising and spending money on amusement in the evening (quoted in Yamamoto 1925: 145–147). A self-denying and determined spirit makes young people useful as both war and company soldiers.

Early Rising and Company Soldiers

The wartime generation was deeply influenced by their participation in the *seinendan* and *gunjinkai*[6]. In later life, they picked up some of the elements of spiritual training to form their own groups and movements. One of them is Maruyama Toshio (1892–1951) who, being deeply concerned about the spiritual fatigue of his fellow countrymen, founded the ethics association in 1948. Its members have written several self-improvement books on early rising. The head of the Tokyo branch, Kawamura Shigekuni (1992: 96–97), explains that the 'goal is to create happy families, cheerful regional societies, and a peaceful international society; every individual member works steadily to achieve a "pure ethic", to realise and spread these principles'.

The association organises training weeks for company employees in which these ideals are put into practice. American anthropologist Dorinne Kondo (1990: 78–104) participated in such a training week. According to her detailed description, all participants were woken by loudspeakers at 5 a.m. the entire week. They had fifteen minutes to get dressed, wash their faces, brush their teeth, make their beds, and make their way to the hall. If one participant did not adjust, the whole sub-group was punished. The individual groups were then assigned cleaning tasks, which they carried out with an enthusiastic *'faittō!'* (*fight!*). That was followed by jogging to the statue of the founder, Maruyama. Upon arriving there, a tape played the *Kimi ga yo*. The *Hi no maru*[7] and the flag of the ethics movement were raised, and after an 'uplifting' morn-

....

6 For sake of brevity, I limit my analysis to the rural youth, as they have received little scholarly attention. However, soldiers and elite students 'enjoyed' a similar training. High schools introduced sport clubs in the late nineteenth century, influenced by both samurai martial arts and Anglo-American high-school and university sports. Club members had early-morning winter practise, *kangeiko*, for which they sometimes started their day at 4.30 a.m. 'Truly we call this manhood', commented a member of the Hachiman Commercial Kendo Club in 1921 enthusiastically (cf. Cave 2004: 386–392). Similar sports clubs are a central element of school life today, and there are also training units before classes start, however, usually a bit later than 4.30 a.m..

7 The *hinomaru*, the white flag with the red sun disc, was first given legal status as the national flag in 1999 and is generally regarded as a national symbol reminiscent of pre-war and war-time nationalism. At the same time, *kimigayo*, which celebrates the thousand(s) of generations of the imperial family, has become the national anthem.

ing appeal (*chōrei*) to the group at the foot of the 'almighty' Mt. Fuji, one of the participants had to explain what his or her impressions were of this speech. The next point on the programme was a shout training, 'good morning, Mrs. so-and-so; thank you, Mr. so-and-so' and, most importantly, 'good morning father, good morning mother'. Next was an approximately two-kilometre run as well as a *misogi* (ritual washing) with ice cold water: sitting on their heels, the washers poured the water down their backs. The next item on the program was the morning meeting. The participants were first allowed to sit down for breakfast at 8.30 a.m.

At the morning meeting, one of the school's representatives held a lecture explaining inspirational sayings such as 'suffering is the gateway to happiness' or 'today is our best day.' Due to hunger and exhaustion, most participants listened only half-heartedly and understood very little of the often complicated explanations. Early rising was the theme of the first lecture: 'This day ... comes only once. Waking up late means standing on the losing side from the start. It is unnatural. And if one gives in to the desire to remain in bed, it leads to egotism, passivity, a disturbance of the bodily rhythm, messiness, mishaps, and, in the end, unhappiness.' Contrary to this, it is 'natural to jump out of bed just after waking. This leads to a loyal, upstanding heart, to positive and constructive behavio[u]r, and to success and happiness' (Kondo 1990: 84).[8]

As in the teachings of *hōtokusha* and *seinendan*, suffering is considered to be a path to overcoming one's own weaknesses and outgrowing inadequacy. The goal is to train an upright, devout, and cheerful heart, which enables one to deal with any upcoming hardship. Chairman Kawamura interprets his own experience by revealing that rising early brings positive energy. Since becoming a member of the ethics association, his business has been extremely successful. Economic conditions were advantageous, but 'I think that it is also related to the fact that I became used to early rising, have become a positive person and in the end full of energy' (Kawamura 1995: 5–6). Since one learns to overcome negative emotions such as laziness and weakness, in the end one becomes forward-looking and grows stronger. Self-control and overcoming laziness are qualities that are valued at the workplace and are often considered

....

8   For a similar training see Rohlen 1973. One famous training is known as the hell camp (*jikoku no kunren*), the Kanrisha yōsei gakkō, run by the Shain kyōiku kenkyūjo (Research Institute for educating employees), which is also connected to the Fuji-san isshōkenmei gakkō (Mount Fuji with-all-your-might-school). Its aim is to 'attach a proper lifestyle and good manners to the body' (*reigi tadashii seikatsu ya aisatsu nado o mi ni tsukeru*). www.shainkyouiku.jp; www.shain.co.jp (incl. videos).

characteristics of the kind of masculinity promoted by the energy drink advertisements quoted above.

The ethics association or movement ties the education of early rising to emotional, *shintō*-nationalist symbols such as flags, hymns, Mt. Fuji, and ritual cleansing and thereby quite explicitly connects early rising with patriotism.[9]

Although in the camp situation the spiritual training by means of early rising and related activities is more concentrated, similar elements are also integrated into everyday work and school life. Morning gymnastics and other sports, individual book reading, morning calls and reading out loud, are often scheduled before the official work or school day begins and are often compulsory. Since 23 October 2003, teachers and students have to stand every morning and sing the national anthem while the flag is raised, a much contested regulation. These activities not only force everyone to get up early, but by following certain routines and rituals, people are meant to prepare gradually for social life. As Catherine Bell (1992: 204) points out, rituals exert a fundamental strategy of power by forcing the expression and internalisation of the values and structures of society as a whole, in and by the body.

In the interview quoted above, Mr. Nagamatsu places sleeping late in the same category as unkempt hair, an unshaven face and informal dress. This is no coincidence: An important part of the daily morning rituals for both men and women has always been to make their appearance more formal, with special emphasis being given to one's hair – as far back as the house code of the powerful Fujiwara family in the tenth century (quoted in Hashimoto 1986: 27–28). As in Nagamatsu's statement, a line in a girl's textbook from the Edo period, the *Onna jitsugokyō*, virtues of early rising, proper hair grooming and the devout performance of one's duties are closely linked: 'Rise early in the morning and comb your hair, serve your father- and mother-in-law' (Kurokawa 1977: 125).

Hair has a distinct symbolic value, and not only in Japan. Hairstyle is indicative of social status. The condition of one's hair reflects the spiritual state of one's mind, and symbolises (male and female) energy and vitality (Muchi 1993: 188). Witches and ghosts are depicted with tousled hair. Hair, as well as the whole body, must therefore be brought under control. Today, even though it is much more common to take a bath in the evening than a shower in the morn-

---

9   This connection can be found in other countries as well, especially in militaries all over the world (cf. Ben-Ari 2003) or in the Hitlerjugend, fascist youth organisations or the Hinduist nationalist movement.

ing, many young women and men wash their hair again in the morning, even if they have to sacrifice breakfast for it (for which they are strongly criticised). At the least, they make use of the various cosmetics available to maintain their hair's proper appearance throughout the day. Bodily hygiene in general and donning a formal uniform emphasise the transition into social life. By the time people start their daily duties, they are prepared to invest them with their positive energy and attitude.

Gendering Early Rising and the Beautiful Japanese

Until recently early-rising books usually addressed men, and even in the 1990s they were authored exclusively by men. Sacrificing sleep is usually seen as a male thing, and the majority of people assume that on average, men get up earlier than women. However, empirically this is not true. According to the NHK time-use surveys, in almost all age and professional groups, on average, women leave their beds or futons about twenty to thirty minutes earlier than their husbands or male counterparts. The only exception is women in their early twenties.

Pre-modern sources indicate that this is not a recent trend. Women – especially when newly married – were always the first to rise and last to go to bed (to have time to care for everybody else). The Confucian phrase 'rise early and go to bed late', stood metaphorically for a woman's piety and devotion to the family into which she had married; and it was not only a metaphor. Tsuboi Kashō reports the following in his *Kawachiya Kashō kyūki*, one of the most important sources describing daily life around 1700:

> *The daughter-in-law makes a pitiable impression. In good as well as bad times, she is always dependent on others. She obeys her husband, is at the mercy of the mood of her father-in-law and mother-in-law, goes to sleep late and gets up early. (Nomura et al. 1955: yome to iu mono wa)*

Gender relations have dramatically changed since this time. But whereas men's work schedules determine the waking time, even today one of women's important duties is to make sure that everyone gets out of bed and the house in time, prepare breakfast for all and healthy lunch boxes for children of kindergarten age and possibly other family members and help children take to school

© Frank & Timme   Verlag für wissenschaftliche Literatur

everything they need. Housewives also hang the futons in the sun so that they will become dry and comfortable, and put them away in the cupboard as crucial preparation for the coming night. They thus ensure the whole family's smooth transition from night to day. Even when women have full-time jobs, they cannot escape this responsibility.

Women's early rising was and still is not associated with a work ethic, social advancement or social responsibility, but instead with filial piety or loving care for her family. Women are meant to support their husbands and families in achieving an honourable place in society, but can not claim the same for themselves. Women's lives are regulated indirectly through the social demands of the public lives of their fathers, husbands and children.

In a typical job as a so-called 'office lady' in a large company, women have duties similar to those they have at home. Laura Kriska (1997: 48–51) describes the women's morning routines in the executive office at Honda company: Well before the official start of work at 8.40 a.m., they have already arrived at the office in their uniforms, cleaned the previous day's dishes, prepared the drinks for the day, dusted off all the tables, put out the working utensils, sharpened the pencils and got to their desks a few minutes before the work bell rings, telling them to start their desk work. It is only at this time that the male executives arrive. Just as at home, women are responsible for men's transformation process into their duties of a *shakaijin*.

Since the 1990s, more and more women have postponed their marriage or do not marry at all and family structures are weakening (Iwakami 2007: 82–85). It has thus become increasingly difficult for (state) institutions and corporations to regulate women's behaviour indirectly through their husbands or children. Women cannot be convinced to get up early to take care of the family if they don't have one. It thus comes as no surprise that the latest trend in promoting early rising addresses women directly by promising that they will lose weight and become beautiful. Oba Shirō (2007) suggests a 'two-minute morning diet to slim beautifully'. The (probably correct) assumption seems to be that while young women increasingly refuse to sacrifice their own goals for husband and children, they are quite willing to make sacrifices to shape their bodies, although the effect of the books might not be long lasting.

Early-rising promoters make an astounding number of references to beauty nowadays. The morning expo of April 2008, for instance, offers a lecture on 'the lips of the beautiful person'. The website suggests that one will become the person one wants to be and invite good luck by moving the lips beautifully.

Mountaineer Tabei Junko presents a lecture on hiking the beautiful Japanese mountains (http://asaexpo.net/2008spring/pro-eccoz.html#04). Early-rising proponents have long advertised the 'beauty of the morning' – preferably in tamed nature – for both women and men. In the 'land of the rising sun', greeting the sun bears additional meaning as a national symbol, as is shown in the early Meiji school textbooks. Beautiful smells are also advertised. While the morning expo offers coffee-brewing classes, women also serve a perfect 'traditional' Japanese breakfast with miso soup. Being woken by 'the smell of miso soup for breakfast', freshly prepared by their wives, has long been idiomatic to describe an ideal marriage and morning; and many men deeply regret that they can no longer expect such a service.

The emphasis on beauty does not alter the underlying moral principles of early rising. On the contrary, the notion of 'beauty' has lost its innocence since Prime Minister Abe Shinzō's (26 September 2006 to 12 September 2007) attempts to encourage patriotism under the slogan of building a beautiful country, a slogan that evokes spiritual teachings rather than political manifestos. And indeed, in 2006 the 'Council to Make Japan Beautiful' (Nihon o utsukushiku suru kai), in co-operation with the Ministry of Education, Culture, Sports, Science and Technology and 150 other organisations including PTAs and pre-school educational institutions launched a contest entitled 'Hayane, hayaoki, asagohan' (early to bed, early to rise, breakfast). People were asked to submit slogans and pictures on the topic to be used for a campaign in 2007. Several children's books promoting early rising and songs with choreographed gymnastics on video have been produced; all over the country pre-schools organise events promoting this lifestyle. The explicit aim is to train children to have a regular rhythm of going to bed and getting up early and having regular breakfast. The website quotes studies showing that children adhering to such a rhythm not only perform better at school, but also 'have shown to have a better sense of morals and justice', thereby explaining the aims of the campaign (www.hayanehayaoki.com, acc. 30 December 2007; the Council to Make Japan Beautiful is no longer on the new website: www.hayanehayaoki.co.jp, acc. 20 February 2008).

On the website of the June 2007 morning expo, the 'hayane, hayaoki, asagohan' campaign is cited as a partner. Thus, these campaigns can be seen as conscious and co-ordinated attempts to integrate as many social groups as possible and spiritually align them into the governments' and business circle's aims to foster self-denial and patriotism. While the morning expo (as well as another campaign called 'morning project', http://www.asa-pro.net), self-improvement books and training camps target male (and increasingly female) *shakaijin*, the '*hayane, hayaoki, asagohan*' campaign is aimed at pre-school children and their mothers.

Conclusion

While sleep is necessary, it bears an anarchist potential for shirking social duties and it is difficult to control. Waking up, getting out of bed, washing, dressing, combing one's hair, eating breakfast, doing physical exercises, preparing work tasks and other routines or rituals present a transition from the private to the social and public spheres. The purpose of this transition is to convey a message about the nature of social requirements and to switch the body from the sleep mode to an attitude that enables appropriate contributions to social life. Therefore, co-ordinating this time with the schedules of wider society and the regulations of morning activities is an important tool for embodying social order (cf. Bell 1992: 97). While men and children are targeted through early-rising campaigns, for the most part, it is women's duty to ensure the whole family's smooth transition from sleep to the performance of social and public activities, and in their roles as company employees women are often burdened with the same responsibilities.

Promoters of early rising promise a bouquet of merits: health, wealth, wisdom, happiness and even beauty. Nonetheless, the key reason for rising earlier is to learn to suppress or control one's emotions, feelings and desires. By overcoming inclinations towards weakness and laziness and dealing with the hardship, one is said to gain positive energy. The method of cultivating the body by means of early rising has been used by religious faiths for centuries. It is a powerful tool to educate people in self-denial and to align them spiritually. In Japan, from the early twentieth century, nation-wide, government-controlled organisations, such as *hōtokukai* and *seinendan*, have worked with early morning activities to increase patriotic sentiments and achieve national goals of economic advancement and military power. It is thus no coincidence that nation-wide initiatives to encourage early rising have re-gained momentum at a time when Japanese leaders have worked towards increasing love for the nation. Although Abe whose slogan of Japan as a beautiful country is reflected in the campaigns stepped back as prime minister in summer 2007, early-rising campaigns continue to prosper.

Bibliography

BELL, CATHERINE (1992) *Ritual Theory, Ritual Practice*. Oxford and New York: Oxford University Press.

BEN-ARI, EYAL (2003) 'Sleep and Night-time Combat in Contemporary Armed Forces. Technology, Knowledge and the Enhancement of the Soldier's Body', BRIGITTE STEGER AND LODEWIJK BRUNT (eds) *Night-time and Sleep in Asia and the West. Exploring the Dark Side of Life*. London: RoutledgeCurzon, 108–126.

CAVE, PETER (2004) 'Bukatsudō: The Educational Role of Japanese School Clubs', *Journal of Japanese Studies* 30(2): 383–415.

FUJIMOTO KENKŌ (1995) *Anata o kaeru chō-'jukusui tanmin'-hō* (The ultra-short-sleep method that changes you). Tōkyō: Mikage Shobō.

HAVENS, T[HOMAS] R. (1983) 'Ninomiya Sontoku', *Kodansha Encyclopedia of Japan*, Volume 6. Tōkyō: Kōdansha, 7–8.

GENDAI JŌHŌ KŌGAKU KENKYŪKAI (1994) *Asa no chiteki seikatsujutsu* (The technique to use the morning wisely). Tōkyō: Kōdansha.

HANI YOKO (2007) 'Spreading the "Early-Bird" Word. In Praise of the Morning's Glory', *The Japan Times* 10 June. http://search.japantimes.co.jp/print/fl2070610x3.html (acc. 11 June 2007).

HASHIMOTO YOSHIHIKO (1986) *Heian kizoku* (Heian aristocracy). Tōkyō: Heibonsha.

ITŌ OSHIRŌ (1972) *Fukuoka-ken shi-shiryō. Dai-6-shū* (Historical sources of Fukuoka prefecture 6). Tōkyō: Meicho Shuppan.

IWAKAMI MAMI (2007) *Raifukōsu to gendā de yomu kazoku* (Understanding family through life-course and gender). 2nd ed. Tōkyō: Yūhikaku.

KAIBARA EKIKEN (1995) *Yōjōkun. Wazoku dōjikun* (Teaching on healthcare. Teachings for Japanese children). Edited by Ishikawa Ken. Tōkyō: Iwanami Shoten.

KAWAMURA SHIGEKUNI (1995) *'Asa' no yutaka na tsukaikata. Un ga kawaru, hito ga kawaru* (A wealthy way of making use of the morning. Fate will change, the person will change). Tōkyō: Sangokan.

KOKUNI YOSHIHIRO (2007) *Sengo kyōiku no naka no 'kokumin'. Ranhansha suru nashonarizumu* (The 'nation' in post-war education. The diffusion of nationalism). Tōkyō: Yoshikawa Kōbunkan.

KONDO, DORINNE (1990) *Crafting Selves: Power, Gender, and Discourses of Identity in a Japanese Workplace*. Chicago: University of Chicago Press.

KRISKA, LAURA (1997) *The Accidental Office Lady*. Rutland, Vermont and Tokyo: Tuttle.

KURIYAMA SHIGEHISA (2002) 'The Enigma of "Time is Money"', KURIYAMA SHIGEHISA UND HASHIMOTO TAKEHIKO (eds) *The Birth of Tardiness: The Formation of Time Consciousness in Modern Japan* (= Nichibunken Japan Review 14): 217–230.

KUROKAWA MASAMICHI (1977) *Kyōkasho-hen* (Textbooks). Tōkyō: Nihon Tosho Sentā (= Nihon kyōiku bunkō 9 [Japan educational library]).

KUROSAWA MASATSUGU (1994) *Asagata ningen de rakuraku shikaku ga toreru. Fukyō-shitsugyō jidai ni jibun o takaku uru totteoki no hōhō* (As a morning person you can comfortably earn qualifications. How you can sell yourself expensively in a time of economic troubles and unemployment). Tōkyō: Jitsugyō no Nihon-sha.

LINHART, SEPP (1988) 'From Industrial to Post-industrial Society: Changes in Japanese Leisure-Related Values and Behavior', *Journal of Japanese Studies* 14(2): 271–307.

MAEDA HIROSHI (1999*) 'Meiji-ki ni okeru "(chūō) hōtokusha" ni kansuru kihonteki shiryō'* (Basic sources on the *hōtokusha* during the Meiji period), *Shukutoku Daigaku Shakaigaku kenkyūjo* 33: 257–288.

MOCHIZUKI [BUKKYŌ DAIJITEN] (1967 [¹1933]) 'Goyoku' (Five desires), TSUKAMOTO ZENRYŪ (ed.) *Mochizuki bukkyō daijiten* [Mochizuki large Buddhist dictionary] vol. 2. Tōkyō and Kyōto: Sekai Seiten Kankō Kyōkai, 1385–1386.

MUCHI YŌKO (1993) *Yume to nemuri no shiyōhō. Motto jibun ga suki ni naru (*How to make use of dreams and sleep. Getting to like oneself even more). Tōkyō: Dōbun.

NHK [HOSŌ BUNKA KENKYŪJO] (several years) *NHK Kokumin seikatsu jikan chōsa.* (NHK national time-use survey). Tōkyō: Nihon Hōsō Shuppan Kyōkai.

NISHIMOTO IKUKO (1997) 'The "Civilization" of Time. Japan and the Adoption of the Western Time System', *Time & Society* 6(2-3): 237–259.

NOMURA YUTAKA ET AL. (1995 eds) *Kinsei shomin shiryō. Kawachiya Kashō kyūki* (Early modern sources on the common people. The Kawachiya Kashō kyūki). Ōsaka: Seibundō.

OBA SHIRŌ (2007) *'Asa 2fun' daietto. Kantan! Kimochi ii! Kirei ni yaseru* (The 2-minute morning diet. Easy! Comfortable! Slim beautifully). Tōkyō: Ōsama bunkō.

ŌMIKA NAOKO (2006) *'"Otona no hayaoki" ga saikin no torendo!?'* (Is there a recent trend in 'adult early rising'?) *All about* 8 November. http://allabout.co.jp/health/stressmanage/closeup/CU2061108/ (30 November 2007).

PYLE, KENNETH B. (1973) 'The Technology of Japanese Nationalism: The Local Improvement Movement, 1900–1918', *Journal of Japanese Studies* 33(1): 51–65.

RAMSEYER, J. MARK (1979) 'Thrift and Diligence. House Codes of Tokugawa Merchant Families', *Monumenta Nipponica* 34(2): 209–230.

RICHTER, ANTJE (2001) *Das Bild des Schlafes in der altchinesischen Literatur* (Images of sleep in early Chinese literature). Hamburg: Hamburger Sinologische Gesellschaft.

ROBERSON, JAMES (2005) 'Fight! Ippatsu!! "Genki" Energy Drinks and the Marketing of Masculine Ideology in Japan', *Men and Masculinities* 7(4): 365–384.

ROHLEN, THOMAS (1973) '"Spiritual education" in a Japanese Bank', *American Anthropologist* 75(5): 1542–1562.

SAISHO HIROSHI (1994) *'Asagata ningen' no himitsu. Shukkinmae no 100nichi kakumei* (The secret of the morning type person. The revolution of the 100 days before going to work), (1st edition 1991) Tōkyō: Jōhō Sentā Shuppankyoku.

SATŌ DEN (2005) *'Asa' nikki de yume o kanaeru nōto* (Notes on fulfilling dreams with the morning diary). Tōkyō: PHP kenkyūjo.

SEINENKAN (1989 ed.) *Dai-Nippon seinendan-shi* (History of Great Nippon seinendan), Reprint (1st ed. 1942). Tōkyō: Seinenkan (Fuji shuppan).

STEGER, BRIGITTE (2004) *(Keine) Zeit zum Schlafen? Kulturhistorische und sozial-anthropologische Erkundungen japanischer Schlafgewohnheiten* ((No) time to sleep? – Cultural history and social Anthropology of Japanese sleep habits). Münster: LIT.

TANI TERUHIRO (1984) *Wakamono nakama rekishi* (History of youth organisations). Tōkyō: Seinenkan (Fuji shuppan).

WU, SARA AND ERIC CHANG (2008) 'The Rise of the Early Birds: Your Future Begins at Dawn', *Common Wealth magazine*, 30 January. http://www.cw.com/tw/english/article/390160.jsp

UJITANI TSUTOMU (1993) *Zengendaigo-yaku. Nihon shoki (ge)* (The Chronicles of Japan). Tōkyō: Kōdansha.

YAMAMOTO TAKINOSUKE (1925) *Hayaoki* (Early rising). Tōkyō: Kibōsha.

YAMASHITA DAIKŌ (1999) 'Rajio taisō to kokumin kokka' (Radio callisthenics and the nation state), THE JAPAN SOCIETY OF EDUCATIONAL SOCIOLOGY (eds) *Nihon kyōiku shakaigakkai daihappyō yōshi shūroku* 51: 93–94.

Authors

Sara Arber is Professor of Sociology and Co-Director of the Centre for Research on Ageing and Gender (CRAG), University of Surrey, UK. At Surrey, she was Head of the School of Human Sciences (2001-04) and of the Sociology Department (1996-2002). She has published extensively on gender and ageing, and health inequalities, and with colleagues at Surrey has latterly pioneered research on sociology of sleep.

Eyal Ben-Ari is Professor in Sociology and Anthropology at Hebrew University of Jerusalem. Previous publications include *Body Projects in Japanese Childcare* (1997) and *Mastering Soldiers* (1998). Among recent edited books are (with Edna Lomsky-Feder) *The Military and Militarism in Israeli Society* (2000), (with Daniel Maman and Zeev Rosenhek) *War, Politics and Society in Israel* (2001), and (with Timothy Tsu and Jan van Bremen) *Perspectives on Social Memory in Japan* (2006).

Emanuela Bianchera is a Marie Curie Research Fellow at the Centre for Research on Ageing and Gender, Department of Sociology, University of Surrey. She graduated from Parma University, Italy, and is currently conducting research for her PhD on gender and care-work in Italy addressing how family care connects with sleep, well-being and work-life balance.

Lodewijk Brunt is Emeritus Professor of Urban Studies at the University of Amsterdam (Netherlands). His research activities led him to study Indian city life, Mumbai's in particular. Of late he has been translating Hindi poets on cities into Dutch and he is preparing a book of Hindi film song translations. With Brigitte Steger he edited *Night-time and Sleep in Asia and the West* (2003, 2006).

Robert Cox is an historian and archivist at the University of Massachusetts, Amherst. He is author of *Body and Soul: A Sympathetic History of American Spiritualism* (2003) and editor of *The Shortest and Most Convenient Route: Lewis and Clark in Context* (2004).

John Dittami studied Chemical Engineering, Biology and Life Science Engineering at Tufts University, Medford, MA. He received his doctorate from the Ludwig-Maximilians-University, Munich, in 1981 and his *venia legendi* from the Eberhart-Karls-University, Tübingen, in 1987. His main research interests are endocrine and neuroendocrine aspects of biological rhythms (circadian and circannual), stress management and reproduction.

Gerhard Kloesch studied Psychology and Political Science in Vienna. He is scientific staff member in the sleep laboratory of the Department of Psychiatry since 1989 and sleep and dream researcher at the Department of Neurology (Medical University of Vienna) since 1997. Since 1993, his research has focused on the clinical application of activity measuring by means of actigraphy for the diagnosis of sleep/wake cycle disorders.

Gabriele Klug earned her Mphil in German and English Studies at the University of Graz, Austria, in 2005. Her book on sleep as a motif in medieval German literature was awarded with the 'Sleep Research-Award 2006 for the Promotion of Young Scholars' by the German Sleep Research Society. Currently, she is doing a PhD in German Studies, receiving a 'Doc-Team' fellowship by the Austrian Academy of Sciences.

Ileen Montijn studied history at the University of Leiden and worked for the Dutch national daily newspaper *NRC Handelsblad*. Among her books are *Leven op stand 1890-1940* (first ed. 1998), about upper class home life in the Netherlands, and *Tussen stro en veren* (2006), about the bed in the Dutch interior.

Brigitte Steger is a Lecturer in Modern Japanese Studies at the University of Cambridge, UK. She has earned her PhD from the University of Vienna, Austria, for her award-winning study on Japanese sleep habits. Her publications on sleep include *(Keine) Zeit zum Schlafen?* (2004) and *Inemuri* (2007, in Braille 2008); with Lodewijk Brunt she edited *Night-time and Sleep in Asia and the West* (2003, 2006).

© Frank & Timme   Verlag für wissenschaftliche Literatur

Susan Venn is a researcher and PhD student at the Centre for Research on Ageing and Gender at the University of Surrey, UK. Susan's research focuses on gender, ageing and the sociology of sleep. She has previously worked on projects investigating the negotiation of couples' sleep, and is currently researching poor sleep among community dwelling older people (SomnIA).

Pia Vogler is a DPhil candidate at the Department of International Development (QEH), University of Oxford, UK. She is currently working on a doctoral dissertation on the daily, seasonal and life course transitions of Karen children in Northern Thailand. Related to her academic interests, she conducted consultancies for the UN High Commissioner for Refugees (UNHCR), the Bernard van Leer Foundation as well as the Young Lives Project (University of Oxford).

Index

actigraph /actigraphy   17, 95, 97ff., 167

age   9, 18f., 22, 79, 83, 93, 97, 108, 111, 113ff., 123f.,
126, 131, 135ff., 147, 157, 171, 178–181, 184f.,
198, 208, 221, 230

agency   180, 194, 208f.

alba   37, 46, 49

alcove   82ff.

alcohol   106, 197, 219f.

animism (see *nat / nats*)

Auping   12, 87–90

awakening   59, 63, 66, 98f., 115, 121, 125, 140, 146

bamboo hut   197f., 200–203, 207f.

beauty / beautiful   40, 42, 45, 61, 138, 159, 163, 211, 230–233

bed clothing (see also
sleep clothing)   10

bedbugs   14, 19, 24, 75, 79

bedding   12, 19, 54, 85, 93, 96, 196f., 199f., 208

bedroom   17, 19–22, 24f., 33, 75f., 78, 80ff., 85ff., 90, 106f.,
117, 119, 121f., 124f., 156, 175, 177–181, 183f.

bedstead   77, 79, 85

bedtime   19, 21ff., 26, 36, 106f., 119f., 175, 177–184, 187,
212

bedtime ritual
(see also sleep ritual)   21, 23, 26, 36, 176f., 182f.

bedtime scenario   177, 179f., 183, 188

blanket   19, 25, 85, 157, 169, 198, 200, 202f.

bodily economy   55f., 58

body   26, 33, 36, 38f., 55–58, 60, 63–69, 132, 180, 203,
207f., 220, 228f., 233

box bed   77–86

boy   19, 21, 24, 80, 108, 124, 159, 163, 166, 179, 199, 203f.

Britain   187

Buddhism   20, 205, 211

Burma   25, 193, 197–200, 202, 205f.

callisthenics (see also gymnastics)	220, 224ff.
carer	19, 132f., 135, 142, 145, 147
caregiving	17, 131–135, 140ff., 144–148
caring role	18, 132f., 139f. 147
castration	22, 24, 36, 40
character of sleep	157
childcare	131, 133f., 142f., 177, 179
childhood	18, 21, 26, 83, 163, 175f., 183f., 186f., 197, 199
children (and sleep)	11f., 14, 17ff., 22f. 25f. 36, 67, 75f., 83f., 88, 90, 97, 106–116, 118ff., 122–126, 132ff., 139–144, 147, 156f., 159, 163f., 168f., 171, 175–188, 198ff., 202ff., 206f., 212, 226, 230–233
Christian / Christianity	20, 33, 37ff., 41, 61ff., 76
chronotype	97f.
circadian rhythm	12, 106, 119
class	18ff., 22, 79, 135, 171, 208
cleanliness	75f., 105, 177
condition	27, 54f., 59, 63, 67, 69, 79f., 84, 97ff., 140, 153, 158f., 194, 197f., 201, 206ff., 228f.
Confucianism	20, 211
consciousness	23, 70, 188, 193f., 206
control	11, 14, 18, 20, 25, 33f., 38ff., 56f., 59, 69, 95, 115f., 120, 122ff., 139, 160, 179f., 182, 193, 205, 212, 218ff., 228f., 233
conversational analysis	135
co-sleeping	9, 13, 21f., 76, 85, 93, 169, 183f., 186, 188, 197ff.
couple-sleep (see also pair-sleep)	93
curtain	44, 77ff., 84f., 198
danger	25, 32, 34–38, 43, 45ff., 50, 59f., 113, 202f., 207f.
daughter	106, 110–114, 123, 135, 141, 144, 157, 161, 204, 230
dawn	213f., 216
daylight	36, 49, 119, 155f., 213f.
daytime	10, 13f., 22f., 37f., 42, 44, 64, 79, 84f. 97f., 106, 125, 171, 184, 196, 200, 203

© Frank & Timme   Verlag für wissenschaftliche Literatur

daytime fatigue /
daytime sleepiness 9f., 97, 138
daytime sleep
(see also napping) 37, 42, 44, 167, 184, 203
death / dead 15, 24, 31, 35f., 38, 44, 46, 50, 53, 59f., 62ff., 67f.,
145f., 163, 206, 212, 221
descriptive 62, 156, 162
devil 25, 34, 36, 48, 60f., 161
diecentrism 16
direct observation (see also
participant observation) 155, 160, 196
discipline 15, 58f. 61f., 70, 86, 105, 162, 166, 178, 206
domestic labour 133
domestic violence
(see also violence) 194, 202, 208
dormitory 24, 38, 199
double bed 85f., 178
drawing 36, 136, 197
dream 13, 15f., 34, 41, 55, 61, 63, 65f., 70, 98f., 109, 137ff.,
156, 206, 216f.
dreaming 55, 138, 207
driving 110–113, 115, 125, 135, 153
early rising 20, 26, 75, 211–218, 220, 222–224, 226–234
early-rising association
(see also *hayaoki-kai*) 212, 216, 220, 224
early morning 20, 119f., 164f., 201, 216, 220, 224, 227, 233
educational level 18
eight hours 21, 27, 105, 107, 170, 215
eldercare 131
embodiment / embodied 180, 193f., 203
ethnographic material /
ethnographic approach /
ethnographic study 136, 193, 195, 197
exploratory 136, 153, 156, 181, 193, 195
family household 115, 144
family life 13, 115, 175, 223

father	33, 93, 112–115, 118, 125, 141, 144f., 161, 171, 184, 228–231
fieldwork	193, 195, 197, 205f.
film	12f. 18, 24, 26, 159, 164
folding bed	84f.
futon	15, 184ff., 230f.
gender	13, 18, 21, 40f., 47, 50, 93, 95, 97, 99f., 106, 108f., 111, 113, 115, 126, 132f., 135f., 147, 157, 166, 179, 196, 198, 202f., 208, 219, 230
ghost (see also spirits)	161, 205ff., 229
girl	13, 19, 21, 36, 40, 45ff., 80, 108, 124, 139, 161f., 179, 199, 203f., 224, 229
globalisation / globalised	26, 154, 178, 186ff.
god / gods	15, 33, 37f., 57–60, 62ff., 66, 68f., 161
grandparents	83, 133, 143f., 184
group sleep	93, 96, 100
gymnastics (see also callisthenics)	26, 224, 229, 332
hayaoki-kai (see also early-rising association)	212, 220
health / healthy	9f., 26, 32, 58, 75, 79f., 88ff., 95, 99f., 105f., 116., 124, 134f., 145, 155, 177, 183, 202, 211, 213, 215, 220, 224, 230, 233
Hindu texts	155, 160
history of sleep	14, 54
homeless	20
household	19, 86, 105, 107, 109, 111f., 115–119, 122, 124ff., 134, 144, 156f., 164, 198–202, 204, 222f.
hōtokusha / hōtokukai	221–224, 228, 233
husband	36, 46, 90, 94, 112, 142f., 145, 157, 164, 171, 198, 203, 206, 230f.
hygiene (see also sleep hygiene)	75, 79, 85ff., 230
hygienic / hygienist movement	20, 75f., 79f., 82, 85–89
identity / identities	21, 47, 63, 179f., 185, 194
idle / idleness	58, 63

income   18, 81, 86, 146, 171
India   15, 17, 19f., 22ff., 26, 54, 65, 69, 153–171, 184, 200,
                                211
indulgence   57, 59, 70, 212
inemuri   10, 12
insomnia   10, 14, 146, 158, 164, 180
interruption (of sleep)   106f., 109f., 113–117, 123, 125, 137, 141
interview   17, 78, 83, 108–114, 122, 124, 131, 136f., 140f.,
                                144, 147, 195, 197, 209, 212, 219, 229
intimacy / intimate   44, 82, 131, 136–139, 147, 157, 175, 178, 186, 188,
                                195, 199, 209
Italian welfare state   131, 133
Italy   17, 19, 24, 131, 133–136, 140, 142, 145, 147, 166
Japan   11, 13, 15, 17, 26, 54, 69, 106, 153, 156, 184–187,
                                195, 211f., 216, 218, 220f., 224, 226, 229, 232f.
Karenni   22, 193, 195, 197, 199, 202–208
key cultural scenario   19, 23, 177, 187
knick knacks (for sleep)   15, 106, 121
knight   18, 33, 39ff., 43, 45–48
leisure   214, 217f.
lifestyle   90, 157, 164, 188, 211, 228, 232
literature   12ff., 17f., 22, 25, 31–37, 39–43, 45, 48, 50, 65, 69,
                                78, 86, 160ff., 164ff., 175, 178, 193, 197, 212f.
longyi   200, 203
man / men   18, 21f., 24f., 33, 36f., 39ff., 58, 60, 62, 64, 66f., 76, 80,
                                85, 99, 111ff., 132, 135, 157, 163, 166, 169ff., 198ff.,
                                202f., 206, 208, 213f., 220f., 224, 226, 229–232
manliness / manhood
(see also masculinity)   40, 47, 227
masculinity (see also
manliness / manhood)   18, 43, 50, 229
marriage   90, 94, 115, 139ff., 231f.
married couple   76, 85, 93, 97, 198f.
mattress   9f., 12, 23, 78, 88f., 101, 171, 184, 200
meaning of sleep   53, 115
medical publication /
medical handbook   75, 212

medical research
(see also sleep research)   11f., 14, 17, 26, 79, 167
medicalisation / medicalise   10, 14, 87, 89, 135
medieval German
literature   31f.
mediterranean   26, 134f., 147f., 153, 166
Middle Ages   17f., 31ff., 35, 38f., 41, 43, 77f.
middle class   19, 23, 26f., 79, 82, 154, 164, 171, 175–179, 185–188
military   11, 226, 233
mind   11, 22f., 34, 48, 53, 55–61, 63f., 67f., 90, 94, 107,
                               113, 117, 120, 140f., 145, 161, 166, 171, 196, 204f.,
                               216, 220, 229
mobile phone   15, 106f., 120ff., 125
monophasic sleep   171
monophasic sleep society   26
moral / morality   20f., 38f., 42, 53, 57, 59, 62, 69f., 75f., 79, 90, 105,
                               135, 215, 218, 220f., 232
morningness-eveningness   97
mosquito   9, 22ff., 198, 200, 202
mother   18f., 22, 93, 96, 106, 109, 111f., 115, 118, 124,
                               133f., 140–144, 146, 162, 164, 169, 177, 179f., 184,
                               186, 198, 228ff., 233
Mumbai   24, 153ff., 157, 159, 162ff., 164, 170f.
nap (see also *inemuri*)   13, 48, 53, 94, 153, 157, 161, 163, 166, 171, 179, 181
napping   10, 12, 14, 67, 94, 96, 165, 171
napping culture   26, 153, 165ff., 170
napping in groups
(see also co-sleeping)   168
nat / nats (see also spirits) 25, 205ff.
negotiation   54, 70, 96, 105, 116, 122, 125f., 181
Netherlands, the   17, 19, 21, 26, 69, 76, 78f., 81, 164
New England   17, 53ff., 57, 59, 62, 69f.
NGO   195f., 200ff.

night	9f., 12, 14–18, 22, 24–27, 35ff., 40, 44, 60f., 63, 68, 70, 90, 94, 97–100, 106f., 109–122, 125, 132, 137–147, 153, 155, 157, 159–162, 164f., 170f., 179, 182, 184, 188, 196, 199, 201ff., 205ff., 213, 216, 218ff., 231
night and sleep	15, 17, 26, 44, 137, 140, 154, 159, 175, 196
night time / night-time	17, 23, 106, 110–113, 122, 132f., 146, 170, 182, 197, 201, 203, 205, 214
night-time sleep	17, 106, 214
nocturnal literacy	16
nocturnal sleep / nocturnal tranquillity	93, 153, 200f., 218
noise	9, 107, 113, 118, 123, 125, 144, 158f., 163, 198, 201
non-academic literature	197
novels (see also literature)	13, 78, 155, 160
oversleeping	38f., 46, 164
pair-sleep	93–101
paramilitary	204
parents' sleep	107, 114, 119
parlour	81
participant observation (see also direct observation)	17, 195f.
patriotism	229, 232
personal space	138f., 141, 146
photograph	87, 90, 109, 124, 155f., 158, 165–171, 197, 225
picture (see also visual material)	9, 17, 49f., 155, 167, 169f., 185, 196, 222ff., 232
pillow	9f., 12, 15f., 168, 200
poetry	32, 49, 160
power	15, 19, 40, 46ff., 50, 56f., 125, 160, 180, 186, 206f., 220, 229, 233
power nap / power napping	9f., 26
pre-industrial society / pre-industrial societies	77, 213
privacy	23, 76, 86f., 168ff., 178, 184f., 196, 199, 203
private space	81, 85, 107, 121f., 158, 177, 181
protection	18, 22, 39, 45f., 193, 195, 197f., 200ff., 205f., 208f.

public	9, 13, 19, 22, 39, 46, 70, 100, 117, 153, 155, 157, 161, 164, 166, 170, 187, 202, 233
public domain	23, 167–170
public sleeping	157, 164, 168, 170
punishment	17, 33, 40, 69, 161
qualitative approach	136
qualitative research method	195
race	18, 68
refugee	18, 22, 24, 193–209
refugee camp / camp	17, 193–197, 198–205, 207f.
release (from pressures)	176
Research Institute for Sleep and Society, Tokyo (RISS)	15
sacrificing sleep	20, 230
security	23, 59, 62, 100, 106f., 111, 116, 124, 177, 180, 193ff., 201, 204, 207ff.
seinendan (young men's association)	224, 226ff., 233
self-denying spirit / self-denial	224, 226f., 232f.
self-discipline	20, 58
senses	38, 53, 55, 57, 59ff., 63ff., 67ff., 180
sexual activity	37, 93, 98f.
sexual contact	95, 98ff.
shakaijin	219f., 231, 233
sibling	22, 36, 96, 107, 116ff., 120, 122, 125, 184, 198
siesta	11, 26, 153, 162f., 165f.
siesta culture	166
silence / silent	16, 159, 166, 196, 201
sin (see also sinful sleep)	33, 49, 60f.
sinful sleep	37, 60
sleep alone / sleeping alone	22, 42, 44, 95, 98f., 159, 182, 184f.
sleep civilisation	26
sleep clothing	175
sleep culture	13, 26, 153, 165ff., 170f.
sleep deprivation	9, 13, 40, 99, 142f., 145, 182, 202, 215, 220
sleep diary / sleep diaries	95, 108, 114, 117f., 120

sleep environment / sleeping environment	21, 93–97, 99f., 105, 109, 119
sleep efficiency	97ff.
sleep hygiene	21, 38, 105f.
sleep interruption / sleep disruption	94, 100f., 107, 109, 116f., 124f., 141, 144ff.
sleep medication / sleep medicine	13, 16f., 146
sleep monster	161, 166
sleep pattern	94ff., 105f., 116, 131, 142, 147, 187
sleep quality	97–101, 120, 131f., 136f., 140f., 144f.
sleep research (see medical research)	9, 11f., 14–17, 22, 94, 96, 117, 136, 153, 167, 171, 212
sleep ritual	25, 177
sleeping and waking	156
sleeping arrangement	19, 75f., 86, 93, 107, 118, 153, 183, 185
sleeping behaviour	19f., 195, 202, 208
sleeping clothes (see also bed clothing and sleep clothing)	203
sleeping custom	175, 186
sleeping in public	164
sleeping mat	200
sleeping place	15, 118, 195, 197, 199f., 203, 208
sleeping together (see also co-sleeping, pair-sleep and couple-sleep)	21, 36, 79, 178, 186
sleepwalking	55, 207
social order	23, 55, 57, 67, 212, 233
social reform	20, 54, 79, 81f.
social status	21, 45, 66, 68, 76, 85f., 90, 166, 183, 216, 224, 229
sociology of sleep	14, 54, 105f., 132, 156
soldier	11, 78, 170, 204f., 226f.
son	39, 110, 112ff., 142, 157, 163, 199
sound	15, 22, 38, 43f., 61, 65, 89, 98, 153, 201 205, 208, 224
space (for sleep)	78, 99, 107, 116f., 122, 177, 184, 196, 198
spirits (see also *nat / nats*)	15, 34, 36, 58, 64f., 69, 168

spiritual	23, 33f., 36f., 49f., 53f., 56–66, 70, 162, 168, 194f., 206f., 227, 229, 232f.
status	18f., 21, 45, 66, 68, 75ff., 82, 85f., 90, 105, 147, 166, 183, 188, 198, 216, 224, 227, 229
supernatural being	201, 203, 205f., 208
Surrey Sociology of Sleep Group	132
sympathy	56f., 68
textiles	77, 154
Thailand	17, 193, 198, 203, 207
time-use survey	175, 216, 230
tired	35, 48, 122, 125, 137, 139f., 157, 197, 219
threat (see also danger)	18, 23ff., 33–37, 49, 54, 59–62, 69, 201f., 205, 212
training camp / hell camp / training week	227f., 232
transition	19, 98, 107, 116, 119, 121f., 126, 147, 201, 208, 212, 218, 230f., 233
twin bed	84–87
unguardedness	59
value	18, 20, 26, 33, 43, 45, 58, 97, 138, 160, 170, 177, 179, 186, 188, 217f., 228f.
Vienna	5, 9, 11, 25, 97, 101, 175, 225
vigilance	55, 59f., 63, 202
violence	34, 182, 194, 202ff., 206ff.
virginity	22, 36, 40, 50
virtue	194, 202, 215, 221, 223f., 229
visionary / visionaries	53, 64f., 67ff.
visual material	212
vulnerability / vulnerable	18, 23ff., 31–37, 39ff., 43, 45f., 49f., 55, 60, 89, 113, 119, 125, 169, 176, 178, 193f., 197, 199f., 202, 206–209
watch-man / watch-men	35, 49f., 62, 196
wealth	86f., 211, 213–218, 233
welfare	19, 24, 111f., 131–134, 145, 147, 186
woman / women	17–25, 36–41, 45f., 48, 50, 75f., 80, 94, 99ff., 106, 111ff., 115, 131–148, 162, 164ff., 169, 201, 203, 206, 220, 224, 229ff., 233

women's employment   134
yoga   26, 160, 162, 211
young people   105–108, 114–126, 183, 193ff., 213, 220, 222, 224, 226f.
youth   162, 193, 202, 204f., 224, 226f., 229

Already published:

Night-time and Sleep in Asia and the West
Exploring the Dark Side of Life

edited by Brigitte Steger and Lodewijk Brunt

foreword by Josef Kreiner; with contributions by Ayukawa Jun, Eyal Ben-Ari,
Lodewijk Brunt, Li Yi, Irene Maver, Chris Nottingham, Peter Rensen,
Antje Richter and Brigitte Steger

First published 2003 by Routledge (£ 75), ISBN 0-415-31850-5

Paperback edition 2006 by *Beiträge zur Japanologie* Vol. 38 (20 €)
Institut für Ostasienwissenschaften – Japanologie, Universität Wien
Campus AAKH, Hof 2, Spitalgasse 2, 1090 Vienna, Austria.
http://www.univie.ac.at/japanologie   japanologie.ostasien@univie.ac.at
ISBN 3-900362-21-1 / ISBN 978-3-900362-21-1

About the book:
The phenomena of sleep and night are experiences that most people take for
granted as a natural part of their daily lives. However, both ideas and practices
concerning sleeping and night-time are constantly changing and widely differ
between cultures and societies. Drawing on case studies from China, Japan,
India, Europe and the USA, *Night-time and Sleep in Asia and the West* discusses:

- notions of sleep and sleeping time
- siesta and napping
- developments of sleep patterns determined by socio-economic changes
- the role of sleep in the life of the homeless and the military
- the relationship between fear and sleep
- night-time behaviour of the young in the 19th and 20th centuries
- sleep, night-time activities and moral teaching

This book suggests that far from being natural phenomena, sleep and night-
time are sites of political struggle between groups as distinct as religious
leaders, school boards and political parties. The essays provide an important
resource for students of Asian and cultural studies and will also appeal to the
general reader.